Money, Marriage, and Madness

The Life of Anna Ott

KIM E. NIELSEN

UNIVERSITY OF ILLINOIS PRESS
Urbana, Chicago, and Springfield

1 2 3 4 5 C P 5 4 3 2 1
♾ This book is printed on acid-free paper.

Cataloging-in-Publication Data is available
from the Library of Congress

ISBN 978-0-252-04314-7 (cloth)
ISBN 978-0-252-08501-7 (paper)
ISBN 978-0-252-05202-6 (ebook)

Money, Marriage, and Madness

SABILITY HISTORIES

eries editors: Kim E. Nielsen and Michael Rembis

Disability Histories explores the lived experiences of individuals and groups from a broad range of societies, cultures, time periods, and geographic locations who either identified as disabled or were considered by the dominant culture to be disabled. Conceiving of disability and disabled experiences broadly and spanning a range of embodiments, the series highlights innovative approaches to disability history that deepen our understanding of the past.

A list of books in the series appears at the end of this book.

As always, and with all, for Maya, Morgan, and Nathan.

Contents

Acknowledgments

BOOKS NEVER HAPPEN ALONE, and the process of *Money, Marriage, and Madness: The Life of Anna Ott* generated lots of gratitude. This is a book I urgently wanted to write on a subject that began as a small detail among many. I appreciate the patience, forbearance, and smarts of all those who have listened to (endured hearing) me speak of Dr. Anna B. Ott for what feels like a very long time. Never before have I dragged as many family members to as many cemeteries on as many hot days as I have done during this book project.

Audience members and commentators at St. Paul's East Side Freedom Library, the American Association of the History of Medicine, the Pacific-Rim Conference on Disability, the University of Erfurt, the University of Toledo, and my very smart students provided thought-provoking questions and commentary. Staff and volunteers at the Chillicothe / Ross County Historical Society were cheerful and knowledgeable. My colleagues in Disability Studies at the University of Toledo are marvelous and prove to me once again that interdisciplinary academic programs make better scholars, both disciplinary and interdisciplinary. The funding generosity of the Friends of the University of Wisconsin Libraries, the University of Toledo, and Duke University's Rubenstein Library enabled pivotal research. Librarians at the Wisconsin Historical Society, the University of Wisconsin, and the Rubenstein Library provided invaluable assistance—particularly Michaela Sullivan-Fowler, Lee Grady, and Rachel Ingold. Skilled archivist Debra Anderson of the University of Wisconsin–Green Bay's Cofrin Library first brought guardianship files to my attention. Anonymous reviewers at *Signs* strengthened this project. Dean Charlene Gilbert of the University of Toledo's College of Arts and Letters cheers on her faculty with admirable skill and genuineness. Portions of this work appear in *Signs* and *Rethinking History*.

My cousins Heidi Marzen and Lynnea Nielsen fed me and provided great company during Madison research trips. Dr. Hossein Elgafy and Dr. Joseph Atallah rebooted my body, provided collegial support, and made work possible. Dr. Lori Rokicki performs bodymind preventative maintenance. The capable Kevin Kostin completed my index. Quinton Babcock, Liat Ben-Moshe, Brenda Brueggemann, Susan Burch, Susan Cahn, Angela Carter, Eli Clare, Linda Curtis, Becky Dale, Ally Day, Jim Ferris, Chelsea Griffis, Adria Imada, Alison Kafer, Stefanie Hunt-Kennedy, Linda Kerber, Cathy Kudlick, Willie McKether, Kathie Nielsen, Ron Nielsen, Katherine Ott (aka, The Other Dr. Ott), Vaskar Pahari (capable of both numerical and cooking magic), Ami Pflugrad-Jackisch, Leslie Reagan, Mike Rembis, Naomi Rogers, and David Serlin provided support of numerous kinds. James Engelhardt is a kind human being, as well as a strong intellect and editor. Susan Burch went above and beyond normal friendship duties. Carmel, Dill, Norma Jean, and Pulga provide entertainment. Nate, Morgan, and Maya keep putting up with me. Most of all, while I tend to dislike sweetie-gushing in acknowledgments, I need to sweetie-gush. Nate makes all things easier.

Money, Marriage, and Madness

Introduction

THE LIFE EXPERIENCES of the woman who became Dr. Anna Barbara Blaser Miesse Ott would have surprised few of her contemporaries, though her life reflects the nineteenth century as few today perceive it. Ott lived in a legal context governing money, marriage, and madness that nearly all nineteenth-century women shared. She benefited from wealth, status, and whiteness, but they did not protect her from the vulnerabilities generated by sexism and ableism. Violence and coercion, coupled with resistance and tenacity, dominated her adult life. Her life story is both profoundly irregular and profoundly unexceptional.

Money, Marriage, and Madness is a story of the medical profession, a woman's wealth and the gendered property laws in which she operated, domestic violence, marriage and divorce, institutional incarceration, and an alleged bank robbery. As a teenager Anna and her family migrated from German-speaking Switzerland to Winesburg, Ohio, in 1834. Her first husband, Jonathan Miesse, practiced as a physician in Chillicothe, Ohio, and upon their divorce she acquired significant financial holdings. During this time she also received medical training. After her 1856 marriage to George V. Ott she moved to Madison, Wisconsin, where she served for nearly twenty years as the only female physician in the region (one of two in the state) and garnered additional wealth. Both marriages ended in ugly legal battles. In 1873 her husband and two local physicians testified to her insanity, as well as her legal incompetency, and Anna Ott entered the gates of the Wisconsin State Hospital for the Insane (also known as the Mendota Asylum). She left when she died in 1893.

Despite what might be considered Ott's historical unimportance, she is not irrelevant. Her life and the stories others told about her life reveal much about the history of marriage and divorce, women's legal precariousness in the nineteenth century, the medical profession of the late nineteenth century, and the lives of those considered insane and institutionalized. This is the biography of a woman heretofore unwritten into history, but a woman whose life mattered and matters. Her life reveals much about power, social structures, and the role of law in nineteenth-century America. I have constructed a biography, an analysis, and large claims about ableism, patriarchy, the messy nature of historical forces, nineteenth-century marriage, and institutional incarceration.

Money, Marriage, and Madness argues that law shapes lives and families, as well as the geographical and conceptual boundaries of a life, and that law itself reflects the power structures of historical periods and places. In the middle decades of the nineteenth century, every U.S. state passed some form of a women's property act, enabling married and single women to own and control their own property, and in roughly the same period passed related legislation enabling women to control their own earnings. Whether during her time in Ohio or Wisconsin or while Ott traveled the Midwest making significant land purchases, these hard-fought legal changes enabled her acquisition of wealth, made divorce far more viable, and allowed her to retain custody of her daughter, Aurelia, after her first divorce.

Additionally, while the criteria for divorce remained limited and strict, the mid-nineteenth-century easing of divorce restrictions profoundly shaped Anna's life. Had she lived fifty years earlier she and her first husband, Jonathan, would never have received a divorce; had she lived fifty or one hundred years later, the criteria for divorce would have been far more lenient. The mid-nineteenth-century marital and property laws advocated by the emerging women's rights movement profoundly determined and deepened the depth of individual control Ott had over her body and goods.

The historiography on nineteenth-century divorce and accompanying legal changes is significant and makes convincing arguments for its uneven and gradual expansion, but that historiography rarely includes intimate looks at the slow and sometimes repeated efforts to dissolve individual marriages. This book includes close views of the dissolution of two marriages, at least one of which involved substantial violence. Unsurprisingly, these were painful, often drawn-out, tumultuous negotiations whose historical documentation and legal narratives were shaped by legal constraints.

Just as *Money, Marriage, and Madness* provides an intimate look at marital dissolution, it also provides an intimate and disturbing consideration of domestic violence. Anna's second marriage followed a nearly textbook formula for domestic violence: separation and isolation from family, the removal of economic resources, and the claim by her husband, George, that he acted only in response to her provocations. In mid-nineteenth-century Wisconsin, Anna, her neighbors, and the courts had few legal options with which to respond. All evidence indicates that George beat her viciously, stole her money, and disparaged her publicly. The meanings and consequences of this violence have a history.

In multiple ways, this biography also adds complexity to scholarship regarding U.S. medical history and reflects the ways by which medical history and the growing field of disability history both overlap and are distinct from each other. Anna Ott served as a physician's wife, a physician, and a patient. She is a part of and inseparable from medical history. She lived her entire adult life imbedded in medical frameworks of expertise, power, privilege, and risk that echoed through all she did. The medical field offered her respectability, status, financial wherewithal, and incarceration.

Historians are just beginning to learn more about the lives of people institutionalized in psychiatric and state hospitals in the United States, especially those incarcerated for long periods of time. Anna Miesse Ott bore two children, survived two tumultuous marriages, and had a professional career before local physicians and her husband determined her insane, institutionalized her, and asked the local court to declare her legally incompetent. Her institutionalization was not the inevitable result of her first fifty-four years of life. Instead, her institutionalization came as the messy result of the purposeful actions of others, her own nonconformity, the vulnerability created by the violence of her marriage, the development of psychiatric institutions by the newly created state of Wisconsin, the growing power of medicine, and the attention generated by the combination of her gender, money, and professional standing. This book reveals Anna's life and the ways others defined her before, during, and after her institutional incarceration. This book argues that diagnoses and prescriptive treatments such as those physicians imposed upon the woman who became Dr. Anna B. Ott are historical concepts with contexts, histories, and significant implications and thus historical agents that do significant cultural work. Diagnoses and prescriptive treatments reflect the world in which they live and work. Diagnoses and prescriptive treatments are never ahistorical concepts removed from culture and place.

The process and rates at which diagnoses and resulting prescriptive treatments are given are gendered, racialized, and class-based, as many scholars have shown. Social structures such as medicine, education, and the law, as well as the individuals who work within them, reflect the power structures of their historical period and place. Scholar Jonathan Metzl, for example, has shown how within simply a few decades schizophrenia went from being a white woman's disease of passivity to a black man's disease of aggressiveness. In other words, the diagnoses with which experts label us and that we receive do not emerge as ahistorical truths given to ahistorical biological bodies, minds, and bodyminds (the inseparable interweaving of body and mind as one entity), including diagnoses as disparate as schizophrenia, ADHD, autism, and prostate cancer.[1] Class-, race-, and gender-based diagnoses can and sometimes do lead to debilitating healthcare disparities.[2]

My purpose is not to suggest that diagnoses simply need to be made accurately and implemented neutrally, and then all will be well. I want to convey the contradictory complexity of diagnosis, particularly the complexity of stigmatized and fraught psychiatric diagnoses. The power to diagnose has frequently led to abuses of that power, and diagnosis sometimes ruins lives. Diagnosis, however, also legitimizes, grants access to resources, can heal or reduce discomfort, and can be liberating. Using the historical example of Anna B. Ott and the words of activist and scholar Eli Clare, I argue, "Diagnosis wields power. It can provide us access to vital medical technology or shame us, reveal a path toward less pain or get us locked up. It opens doors and slams them shut."[3]

Diagnosis is a profoundly powerful act of consequence, an act performed by human beings within complex social structures that, in the case of Dr. Anna B. Ott, resulted in the (re)writing of her life story—her past, her future, and how she would be remembered. When others understood Anna as a learned physician, her acts of diagnosis conferred status and financial rewards. When others understood her to be insane, their diagnosis resulted in confinement and isolation. An insanity diagnosis made the later stories of a bank robbery and architectural oddities possible and erased stories of her professional career, activism, and financial gain. Diagnoses' supposed scientific and thus value-free neutrality erased or covered over the possibility that politics, power, money, and gender hierarchies might influence perceptions of Ott's behaviors, success, and riches. Receiving a stigmatized psychiatric diagnosis meant that she could no longer be the diagnostic physician herself (the diagnoser) but could only receive the diagnostic expertise of others (the diagnosee). By diagnosing Ott as manic, physicians and her husband contained her and her life story—literally and metaphorically—in the asylum.

Once she had been determined incompetent and diagnostically in need of institutionalization, Anna lost the legal right to determine where and how her funds were spent. She lost the legal right to come and go as she pleased. From then on, she was confined to the insane asylum except for isolated day "outings," and she could be confined to a space as small as a coffin under the guise of medical treatment. The woman who had only decades previous traveled throughout the Midwest and Europe by herself could no longer leave the building, and sometimes simply her ward, without permission.

In the past decades, scholars have paid increasing and widely varying attention to the historical processes and experiences of institutionalization, frequently arguing about the motivations and social forces that drove the rise of asylums and the professions that developed within them.[4] This book moves in a different direction, seeking to situate and analyze the lives of people who spent time in psychiatric institutions before, during, and after their period of institutionalization.[5] Who were they? In what relationships and communities did they live? What impact did institutionalization have on the arc of their lives? What social forces propelled, and resisted, their institutionalization? What other possibilities existed, or failed to exist, and why? How did their institutionalized and noninstitutionalized lives interact and affect one another? Biography uniquely allows close examination of these questions. By tracing Ott's life before her institutionalization, I seek to contextualize her, situate her in her multitude of relationships, and remind us that institutionalized peoples have and had lives outside asylum walls. By tracing Ott's decades of institutionalization, I have sketched, in varying degrees of detail, an understanding of daily life in a late nineteenth-century asylum and the permeability of its walls. Tracing the stories told of her after her death enables analyses of the impact of the diagnosis of mania and institutionalization on our memory of her.

In the Wisconsin State Hospital for the Insane, as in all institutions, employees and those institutionalized lived daily lives in relationship with one another and with people outside the hospital's geographic boundaries. The relationships, resources, privileges, and oppressions that shaped one's life before institutionalization followed one into a psychiatric institution, permeated one's daily experiences of institutionalization, and remained with one once released (either alive, considered cured or simply hopeless, or dead). I seek to consider institutionalization and daily institutional life not as a time and space apart from but as a time and space profoundly and intricately interwoven with those outside of the institution's geographic and temporal boundaries.

My analysis employs ableism as an analytical tool, though certainly not as the only analytical tool. For those unfamiliar, an explanation. Ableism as a concept and term includes but also goes beyond discrimination against people with disabilities. For example, just as sexism includes but is not limited to laws and policies that restrict women's options, so does ableism include but is not limited to laws and policies that restrict the options of people with disabilities. Just as cultural representations of criminality often reflect racism, so does the near exclusion of people with disabilities from popular culture (except as murderers in horror movies) reflect ableism. Just as housing covenants and loan policies have historically excluded Jews from many neighborhoods, so have funding policies that only support people with disabilities if they live in institutions manifested ableism. And just as homophobia justifies personal and structural violence, so has and does ableism. Ableism permeates all. As Dan Goodley has written, "We have internalised ableist values into the very heart of our ontological souls."[6] Diagnosis in and of itself is not inherently ableist; nor, more specifically, is a psychiatric diagnosis inherently ableist. However, ableism is forcefully present when human beings who receive a diagnosis are stigmatized, isolated, and rendered illegitimate and when their futures are dismissed as void of all good possibility due to their diagnosis.

Ableism is not separate from nor does it trump other analyses or power structures. Structures of power, as well as individual human beings, reside *together* in historical contexts—sometimes seamlessly, sometimes uneasily, and sometimes messily.[7] Anna Ott's life, unsurprisingly, reflected the time and place in which she lived. That time and place constituted and relied on multiple and interlocking power structures. Ableism, patriarchy, US settler colonialism, the privileges of money, and varying other power structures were woven together to create the nest in which Ott and those around her lived their lives. This messy nest includes large structural forces, the vagaries of individual lives, and the interactions of the two. The systems incorporated into intersectional analyses influence interpersonal relationships and individual lives, but the anger, love, and mundaneness of relationships are not only about social forces. For example, patriarchy and money influenced Anna and George Ott's marital relationship, but the reason for its tumultuous nature went far beyond patriarchy and money to include daily details, pain, love, and hopes. Embracing this messiness (as analysis and content) bolsters intersectional analyses, for it is a reminder that identity categories, social structures, and the interplay between them have daily and personal consequences. When deployed by scholars, intersectionality too often focuses on identity categories to the exclusion of the systems that create, reinforce, and justify those categories via interactions both mundane and momentous. Identity categories cannot contain our full stories, and when we mistakenly focus only on categories we as scholars can easily blur or erase lived experiences.

Money, Marriage, and Madness is also a book about the process of uncovering the past and the process of building the uncovering of the past. Scholar Saidiya Hartman has asked, "Is it possible to exceed or negotiate the constitutive limits of the archive?"[8] Anna Barbara Blaser Miesse Ott left behind no words of her own, no personal material goods, and no family anecdotes told down the generations discoverable by me. Instead of the personal memoirs and letters historians often seek, the remaining evidence of her life is in the medical, legal, and financial records others left *about* her. Or, as Michel Foucault wrote about "obscure men," her existence "comes down to exactly what was said about her."[9] These are the evidentiary equivalent of ambiguous echoes: her desires and actions only after they had rippled through the lives, legal actions, and professional aspirations of others, her desires and actions only after they had rippled through powerful social institutions.

I wish to emphasize that the limited nature of my archive of historical sources is not an accident. The marital, legal, and medical structures in which she and those around her lived limited the evidence that remains regarding her. These are structures people created, benefited from, and pushed against. Whether through interrogating archives, reading against the grain, or examining sources up front, I seek to stretch, to pull at, and to examine the margins of their archival limits. I analyze sources not just to acquire their knowledge and content but also to mull over their influence in the historical record. Some of them generate more questions than they answer. I will prod these sources for the stories they hide, the people they erase, the details baked invisible but apparent in the seasoning, and the powers glossed over.

The very legal processes that created legal and stone walls around Anna Ott for the last twenty years of her life generated the limited paperwork by which I first stumbled onto her life. In the initial stages of a project on adults placed under guardianship, I found her file—but as simply one, and not a large one, of over two hundred such files from Dane County, Wisconsin. The file caught my attention because of Ott's status as a moneyed female physician, a not-unheard-of but unusual individual for the late nineteenth century. A good historian is a stubborn detective, and I dug further. The financial consequences of her marriages and numerous divorce filings and her medical career allowed me to follow her trail. Her twenty-year institutionalization provided scant but vital medical records and a cemetery in which to be buried. Amid a pile of historical sources I found an intriguing thread, pulled at it, traced another, then another, and then another. Eventually I even discovered that Ott's son-in-law lay buried only a few miles from my home.

This will be, borrowing the words of historians Hannah Joyner and Susan Burch, a "silhouette biography" rather than a colorful and substantive portrait. None of the ways by which Anna B. Ott entered, leaked, or stormed her way into historical archives was direct. She left legal footprints, but prints shallow enough to convey only that she was there. Others left their impressions of her, their diagnoses of her, their legal claims about her, their legal claims for her. She—her words, her motives, her desires, her being, even her physicality—was, and remains, excluded from the historical archive. As this book will argue, that is not the result of simple chance. Her archival exclusion is the result of a messy pile of events, time, and oppression, of marital violence, divorce, ableism, and decades of familial isolation, followed by twenty years in an insane asylum. Her archival exclusion contributes to her historical erasure and the historical erasure of generations of institutionalized people.

What limited primary sources remain resulted from the late nineteenth-century expansion of legal and governmental structures. The structures resulting from state-building created the women's property laws that allowed Anna to control her own funds and the county courts, whose rulings could take such control away. The emerging bureaucratic state loosened divorce criteria but offered no guarantee of marital happiness or an escape from violence. It built expansive state institutions into which those diagnosed as insane could be contained; the medical, legal, and police processes by which one could be contained; and the recourses by which Anna could have appealed her institutionalization and incompetency. Its structures and policies developed in relationship with the organizations, training, and policies of late nineteenth-century professional medicine. All of these structures both benefited and restricted Ott's daily life.

While claiming to know all is, admittedly, tempting, I do not know everything about Anna Barbara Blaser Miesse Ott. Indeed, there are ways in which I know very little. This may frustrate the reader. All I can do is express sympathy, for every missing piece has been even more frustrating for me. Some of the evidence from which I craft this story can be interpreted in multiple ways, some evidence is contradictory, and some leaves large, unsatisfying holes. Some of the primary sources, I believe, are full of lies. All I and other scholars can do is be honest about the process. My conjectures, I hope, are transparent, just as, I hope, are the evidence and analyses underlying them.

Finally, there are issues of names.

As is nearly always the case when a historian writes about a US woman who married, names are slippery. Born Anna Barbara Blaser in 1819, my historical subject became Anna Barbara Miesse at the time of her first marriage in 1837. Upon her second marriage in 1856 she became Anna Barbara Ott and claimed the title "Doctor." The name by which I refer to my subject will change as we move through her life story, reflecting the changes in her life. The newspaper advertisements Ott purchased about her medical practice referred to her as Dr. Anna B. Ott and are one of very few historical incidents

I have of her stating her own name. Thus, that is the name I will use when referring to her more generally.

Second, and a decision of more substance but less obvious, I refer to Dr. Anna B. Ott by name. Historians and other scholars who write about institutionalized people sometimes use pseudonyms due to the private and coerced nature of the historical records. Because so much of this story takes place outside the insane asylum, based upon evidence from outside the asylum, and from which Anna could be easily identified, I have chosen not to use a pseudonym for her.[10] When referring to specific individuals institutionalized alongside her I use pseudonyms.

Table 1. A Brief Timeline of Dr. Anna B. Ott's Life

1819, April 11	Anna Barbara Blaser was born in Bern, Switzerland
1834, July 31	Ulrich and Barbara Blaser family arrived in New York City
1837, May 23	Anna Blaser married Jonathan Miesse
1838, December 5	Cornelius F. Miesse born to Anna and Jonathan Miesse
1849	Jonathan Miesse filed for divorce from Anna Miesse and later withdrew the petition
1853, March 23	Jonathan Miesse gave $3,000 to Anna Miesse (a likely marital separation agreement)
1855, September 4	Jonathan Miesse filed for divorce from Anna Miesse
1856, March 7	Minetta Minona Ott born to George V. Ott and unclear mother
1856, March 15	Divorce granted to Jonathan and Anna Miesse
1856, May 10 or 11	Anne Miesse married George Ott
1856, November 6	Jonathan Miesse married Elizabeth Kennedy (born 1833)
1858 December–1859 January	Anna Ott filed for divorce from George Ott
1859, February 11	Anna Ott withdrew the divorce petition
1868, December	Anna Ott filed for divorce from George Ott
1870, December	Anna Ott withdrew her 1868 divorce petition
1873, May 12	Anna Ott admitted to the Wisconsin State Hospital for the Insane
1873, September 5	Dane County Probate Court placed Anna Ott under legal guardianship
1881, June	George Ott filed for and received a divorce from Anna Ott
1885, June 3	First medical record of Anna Ott having what state hospital physicians described as a stroke
1893, March 11	Anna Ott died

1. Mrs. Anna Miesse, Local Doctor's Wife

OBSCURITY AND UNREMARKABLENESS marked the early life of the woman who became Dr. Anna B. Ott and whose tombstone sits in the cemetery of the former Wisconsin State Hospital for the Insane. Her first entries into the historical record note only her unexceptionalism: a young body among hundreds of thousands of bodies moving from Europe to the United States and another young woman marrying another young man. Never would I or anyone else have sought her out had I not found the file. The file, only one among many, was not really even a file. Like all the others, it was a folded pile of papers, yellow with age, falling apart, hard to unfold, and bound together by string. Its discovery didn't merit the word *discovery*. There was no magic spark, no smoking gun, no flashing red sign indicating that between its lines, following its invisible threads backward and forward, lay something that might matter. Thus, even the file signified nothing. Once fitfully unfolded, Anna Ott's file spoke to me, a historian of US women and disability, only due to its subject: a mid-nineteenth-century female physician of property and means declared legally incompetent and institutionalized in an insane asylum.

But that's getting ahead of the story.

The remarkableness of Dr. Anna B. Ott is her unremarkedness and unremarkableness and what those two indicate about US history and the methods by which we discern and relay it. While hers is a story easily sensationalized, the individual and structural violence, patriarchy, ableism, and privileges with which she lived are disturbingly normative and familiar.

As it did for so many white women of the nineteenth century, marriage launched the young white woman into adulthood and reframed her legal standing. Marital status defined her. By marrying twenty-year-old Jonathan Miesse in 1837, eighteen-year-old Anna Blaser moved from the home of her parents to that of her husband, changing her name along with her residence, and in the process became a local doctor's wife, a status with its own duties, expectations, and respectable social standing. Marriage redefined her legal and everyday relationship to financial resources. While marriage altered the legal rights and obligations of men little, for women, particularly white women, its impact cannot be exaggerated. As historian Hendrik Hartog stated, "it was the transformation of a single woman into wife that defined marriage in antebellum America."[1]

Marriage, specifically, marriage to a respectable local doctor, conferred upon Anna already determined time demands, social ideals, and responsibilities. By the 1830s canals and railroads had begun to spread across Ohio, and white settlers had killed or driven out longtime indigenous residents. The state claimed several cities with growing industries. Though a free state, Ohio bordered the slave state of Kentucky and maintained a relatively strict system of racial separation. Neither the Blaser nor the Miesse family was made up of poor immigrants who struggled to make a living in factories or mines, as domestics, or as either urban or rural transients. Both families owned property, and many of the men claimed learned professions. All evidence indicates that Anna spoke English and was literate. Whiteness, class, marital status, and gender shaped others' expectations for Anna's life.

The ideals Anna encountered were exemplified and reinforced in Catharine Beecher's *Treatise on Domestic Economy*, a widely popular book reprinted every year from 1841 until 1856.[2] Beecher and much of her famous abolitionist family lived in Cincinnati at this time, and it is probable that Anna either knew of or owned the book. Whether she did or not, a woman of Anna's standing would have felt "the responsibilities of domestic life" and the weight of the ideals described by Beecher. As Beecher wrote about American women, "No women on earth have a higher sense of their moral and religious responsibilities, or better understand, not only what is demanded of them, as housekeepers, but all the claims that rest upon them as wives, mothers, and members of a social community."[3]

The narrative of Anna Barbara Blaser's life before her 1837 marriage is brief and provides no hints as to her character, education, joys, or traumas. The evidence leaves me, as a biographer and storyteller, the void of what scholar Carolyn Heilbrun called "women's storylessness."[4] The substantive evidentiary story of Anna's life began with her legal attachment to a man via marriage. Born in 1819 as the second of thirteen children and the eldest daughter, she likely spent much of her childhood helping with her younger siblings and the household labor. Records from her second marriage indicate that she received a formal education while a child but do not specify its length or content.[5] In 1834 her parents, Ulrich and Barbara Blaser, left the German-speaking town of Langnau, Switzerland, and migrated with their ten children, ages one to seventeen, to the United States. Anna was fifteen at the time of the lengthy and onerous ocean voyage. The two parents bore three more children after they purchased and settled on two hundred acres of land near Winesburg, Ohio.[6] This small amount of information raises more questions than it answers, and again the sparse historical records are limiting. What was included in Anna's education? Did she like to read, play outside, or make friends? We don't know if she was a pleasant child or a difficult young girl, or if she was simply too busy laboring to leave evidence of her personality. Perhaps she considered marriage a welcome release from family obligations. What compelled Anna is a frustrating void; instead, we see only the outlines of historical forces acting upon her and in which she maneuvered.

Anna married Jonathan Miesse three years after her immigration to the United States. He must have been a fine catch. In the late 1820s the future groom had left a German American community in Pennsylvania and settled in Ohio with his brothers, Samuel, Gabriel, Heinrich, and Benjamin. All five brothers bought substantial land in the area upon their arrival. Jonathan's choice of profession and move to Ohio indicates ambition and a desire to advance himself. The simultaneous move of the five brothers from Pennsylvania to Ohio indicates family ties and a desire to sustain them. Three of the five brothers, including Jonathan, had apprenticed as physicians.[7] The marriage of Anna Blaser and Jonathan Miesse took place in the spring, on May 23, 1837. Perhaps Anna held a bouquet of spring flowers at the ceremony, lilacs or irises. It is likely that both bride and groom had relatives at the event, for Anna's family was large, and Jonathan's brothers lived nearby.

In pragmatic terms, the marriage was a good match because Jonathan had the potential to create a relatively lucrative profession and Anna was pregnant. How she and Jonathan met, how they courted, where and how often they sneaked off to have sex, and whether they had intended to marry before learning of the pregnancy are details unknown to me, but by the time of their wedding she was approximately two months pregnant. Even this premarital pregnancy, however, is relatively unremarkable. Unless the couple did not marry, few in the community would have considered the premarital pregnancy highly scandalous, and the pregnancy had no negative professional implications for Jonathan. In December 1837, seven months after the wedding, newly married Anna delivered Cornelius F. Miesse.[8]

As a local medical man, did Jonathan deliver his firstborn son? Did either of his medical practitioner brothers? By the time Cornelius was born, Anna's mother had already given birth to at least ten children. Perhaps the new grandmother, who knew much about childbirth, either delivered or helped with the delivery of her eldest daughter's first child. The newborn Cornelius was less than a year younger than his grandmother Blaser's latest child and would be older than at least two of his mother's siblings. Sometime in 1838 Anna, Jonathan, and their young son moved to the small town of Adelphi, Ohio (twenty miles north and slightly east of Chillicothe), where Jonathan opened a medical practice.[9]

Jonathan must have done well for himself financially, for in 1843 he purchased 12.5 acres on the outskirts of Chillicothe in order to build a new home for his family and expand his medical practice. Chillicothe was an ideal spot for an ambitious doctor and his wife. In the 1840s Chillicothe was a well-established settler community that had by then driven out its original Shawnee residents. From 1803 to 1816 the town had served as the state capital (except for a brief period from 1810 to 1812), and in the 1840s lawyers, lawmakers, and business leaders still strode the streets frequently. Agricultural producers and cattle processors depended on railroads and the Ohio Canal to transport goods to market easily, quickly, and relatively cheaply.[10] The town's widely known and quite large local choral societies added a note of sophistication to the bustle of production.[11] The Scioto River ran through town, surrounded by rich farmland.

The rapidly growing German immigrant community created cultural spaces familiar to both Jonathan and Anna. By 1840, 10 percent of Chillicothe residents were German immigrants, and by 1850 German immigrants constituted nearly one-third of the town's population.[12] A German-language newspaper began in 1849.[13] German Catholics dominated the community, though varying Lutheran worship groups existed. As Anna's father is noted as one of the founders of the German and Swiss Lutheran church in Winesburg, Ohio, and since at least one of her brothers became a Lutheran minister, perhaps she felt more at home in the smaller Lutheran communities.[14]

In addition, a small but visible number of free African Americans had settled in Chillicothe. Nearby, six miles northwest of the town, lay the Stillguest Settlement, founded around 1800, a community of free black farmers who participated in the Underground Railroad. Chillicothe lay fifty miles up the Scioto River from the Ohio River, which separated Ohio from the slave state of Kentucky and served as a primary escape route. Harriet Beecher Stowe's *Uncle Tom's Cabin* (1852) focused national attention on the river. Blacks in Ohio could be required to provide proof of their freedom at any time and

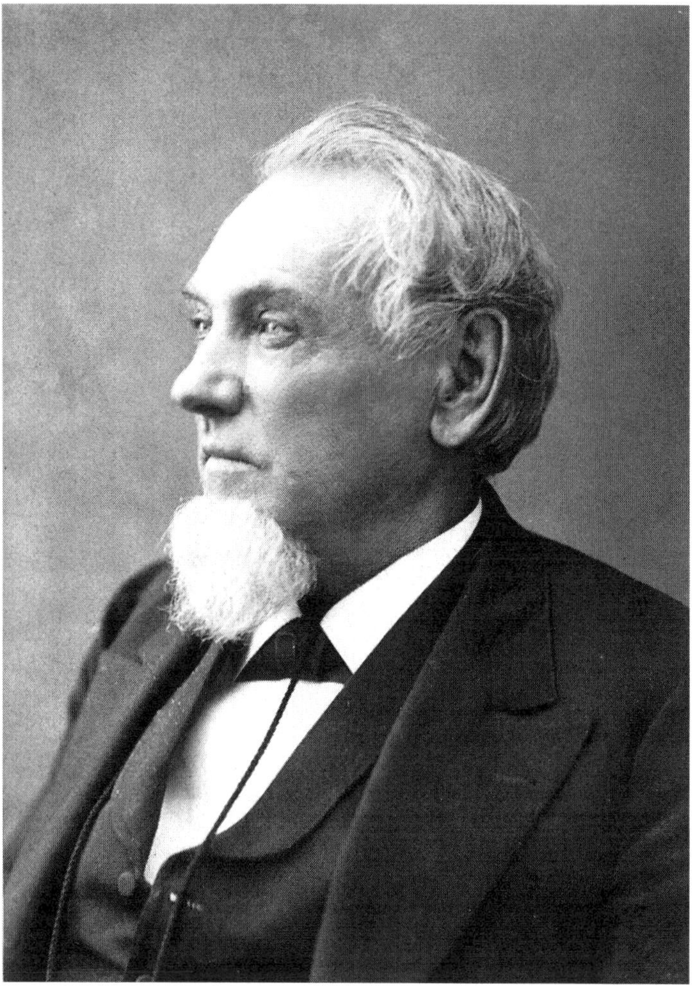

Image 1. Dr. Jonathan Miesse. Courtesy of Ross County, Ohio Historical Society.

had to "post bonds and register with the local county court upon entering the state."[15] Black children were denied public education. Ohio had been a free state since its 1802 constitution, but by the 1830s it was a "white man's republic," and the existence of slavery shaped its politics and daily life.[16]

The status, the privileges, and the labor of being a local doctor's wife, in all of its forms, permeated all of Anna's days in Chillicothe. The home built by Dr. Jonathan Miesse in 1843 was a stately two-story building with a beautiful wooden staircase. Very near the banks of the Scioto River, the house lay removed from Chillicothe and on the other side of the river but close enough to the town for relatively easy access. A bridge and several small ferries made river crossing easy. Perhaps the Miesse household had its own rowboat, to be used for shopping or visiting patients.[17]

The level of Jonathan's training impacted Anna's labor and financial wherewithal. Like most doctors of this period, Jonathan received his initial medical training by serving as an apprentice (usually for a relatively brief period) to an experienced physician. As a community historian put it in the 1880s, Miesse "by private tuition . . . had fitted himself for successful practice."[18] By the 1830s, most states, including Ohio, had societies of medical practitioners, which advocated professional standards and licensing, but Ohio doctors still practiced unregulated.[19] For medical practitioners such as Miesse, the surest way to attain additional legitimacy and prestige was to earn a degree from one of the growing number of medical schools emerging across the nation. To Miesse's advantage, the center of US medical training was Philadelphia. Given his upbringing and initial medical training in Pennsylvania, it was possible that he knew physicians working with one of the emerging Philadelphia medical schools.[20]

In the fall of 1844, with at least ten years of practice under his belt, Jonathan and his brother Benjamin enrolled in the Medical Department of Pennsylvania College, a Philadelphia medical school in operation from 1840 to 1861.[21] With thirty-four other men, the two brothers began their formal studies in early November and continued until early March during the academic years 1844–45 and 1845–46 (two five-month sessions). The Medical Department of Pennsylvania College required its male graduates to attend two sessions of course lectures and complete some clinical instruction.

Upon completing these requirements and writing his thesis on "rheumatismus," Jonathan graduated with an M.D. degree. The Medical Department of Pennsylvania College marked the event with a ceremony at the Philadelphia Museum. The March 5, 1846, event purportedly "attracted a large audience, the principal part of which was ladies," and included music, an opening prayer, and a valedictory address by one of the six professors.[22]

It is unclear if Anna sat proudly among the crowd of ladies attending Jonathan's graduation and if she joined Jonathan for his two five-month academic sessions in the city, increasingly famous for its medical schools. She may have stayed at their new home in Chillicothe with Cornelius to manage the household and possibly maintain some of Jonathan's practice, perhaps relieved not to be with Jonathan or perhaps angry to be left to manage the household for two winters in a row. Jonathan's brother and fellow student Benjamin, who lived not far from them in Ohio, also was married and already had at least one child. Perhaps the sisters-in-law stayed in Ohio while the two brothers lodged together in Philadelphia. If so, perhaps the women traveled together to Philadelphia for the Miesse brothers' graduation. Among all of these unknowns is the clear fact that Anna and Jonathan conceived another child not long after his graduation. Just over nine months later, on January 18, 1847, Anna bore their daughter, Aurelia Carolina Miesse.[23] Cornelius was eight years old.

Whatever Anna's engagement with Jonathan's medical school education, his medical practice shaped the daily routines and labor of her life and that of the entire household when he returned to Chillicothe with an official medical degree. Jonathan would have spent much of his time within the domestic sphere of his family's Chillicothe home, for a midcentury physician saw patients at his home, as well as visiting the homes of his patients. By the turn of the century, medicine would become a full-time, office-based profession, but in the 1840s and 1850s Jonathan likely engaged in multiple means of making a living.[24] He needed a good horse, leather traveling bags, clothing that would keep him warm and dry in all weathers, and medical equipment such as a good knife, candles, and basic drugs. Anna would have worked as receptionist, nurse, and surgical assistant and would have helped to maintain his medical supplies, perhaps even manufacturing medicines—whatever Jonathan needed. Community members easily recognized her as a doctor's wife, perhaps even asking for her medical advice while she shopped, ran errands, or attended community events.[25]

Hard work and a bit of chaos dominated the household and were a part of Anna's domestic routine as the local doctor's wife. Jonathan could be called out to treat a patient at any time of day, and patients showed up at the house unexpectedly. It was Anna's duty to respond, even to triage, if he were unavailable. The household's land along the Scioto River needed planting, tending, and harvesting and likely included various farm animals requiring care. The two growing children required food, clothing, and monitoring. Cholera epidemics periodically swept through Ross County (of which Chillicothe was the county seat), as they did during the summers of 1847, 1848, and 1849, and always held the potential to leave numerous dead in their wake.[26] A major fire hit Chillicothe in April 1852, and Jonathan fought the fire from the roof of a local building and then likely treated burn victims.[27] Besides Jonathan, Anna, Cornelius, and Aurelia, the household variably included multiple others. The 1850 census recorded that two paid laborers lived in the household—one male, one female—as did Anna's eighteen-year-old sister,

Sophia. The assistance provided by the additional adults must have made the household labor easier for Anna and indicates that the couple had the financial wherewithal to pay them.

If we end the story here, Catharine Beecher, the nineteenth-century diva of domesticity, would have approved greatly.

This, however, is where the story gets messy. The household of this small-town physician and his wife, the household in which the children, Cornelius and Aurelia, grew, was complicated, unhappy, and sometimes ugly. Jonathan filed for divorce in 1849, after twelve years of marriage, but withdrew his application within two months. He attempted a separation agreement in 1583. He again filed for divorce in late 1855.

The "open rupture" of the Miesse marriage, as one of Jonathan's legal complaints characterized divorce, was made easier by changing mid-nineteenth-century Ohio divorce laws. In the decades prior to the Civil War, Ohio was known as a "divorce haven" to which many traveled for a relatively easy divorce. In 1850, for example, the state granted one hundred divorces. While that may not seem like many, Pennsylvania, the state's geographical neighbor, had taken the previous thirty-two years to grant that many divorces.[28] An Ohio divorce came easy in comparison to many other states, but criteria remained limited and strict. The acceptable legal grounds were impotency, bigamy, adultery, desertion, habitual drunkenness, fraudulent contract, imprisonment, and "total of gross neglect of duty."[29]

Unfortunately, the records from the 1849 divorce application do not remain and are referenced only in Jonathan's 1855 application for marital dissolution. There Jonathan stated that he had always been a "provident, liberal, faithful, and affectionate husband," but due to his wife's "passionate and quarrelsome character and disposition," he had "lived unhappily" for the first twelve years of marriage (from 1837 to 1849). By 1849 "her course of conduct" had become "so insupportable" that he moved to dissolve the marriage.[30]

Anna apparently did not want the 1849 divorce. A divorce would have left her legally and financially precarious. According to Jonathan, she promised "almost every day" to "reform her conduct towards him, and treat him kindly in future." Jonathan accepted her purported promises and "abandoned" his application, though without the result he desired. He later claimed that within weeks of dropping his 1849 divorce complaint Anna "became again turbulent, quarrelsome, and grossly neglectful of her duty" to himself and the children.[31] "Grossly neglectful of duty" was an important legal phrase, for it served as a legal ground for divorce. Sometime before 1850 Anna's much younger sister Sophia moved into the household and likely left at the time of her 1852 marriage. Did Sophia's presence and then her absence ease the Miesse marital discord or complicate it? Jonathan's version makes no mention of his young sister-in-law.

In March 1853, when Cornelius was fifteen and Aurelia six years old, Jonathan attempted the alternative strategy of a separate maintenance agreement: an unofficial separation bolstered by a financial settlement. At this time, separate maintenance agreements appealed to many couples, and perhaps to the small-town doctor Jonathan Miesse, because of their privacy. Such agreements also meant that a couple could skirt the legal requirement for divorce that one of them be found publicly guilty and the other innocent. This strategy was not unusual; indeed, it was more common than divorce. As historian Hendrik Hartog has noted, "Between 1790 and the middle of the nineteenth century, couples across America separated" without divorce and created their own contracts, verbal or written, about "support, obedience, domicile, custody, and property."[32] A divorce meant, as historian David Silkenat has said about North Carolina marital dissolution in this period, "public and private condemnation from their community" and the public examination of private lives.[33] The details and causes of a maintenance agreement remained private.

Because separate maintenance agreements were private agreements, however, documentation generally was not entered into court records. In this case, financial documents provide the evidence. On March 23, 1853, their sixteenth wedding anniversary, Jonathan gave Anna $3,000—"as a part," the later 1855 divorce petition explained, "of her interest" in Jonathan's estate. Anna could own this property in her own right because Ohio had passed its first Married Women's Property Act less than a decade earlier.[34] Anna presumably received the $3,000 in exchange for releasing Jonathan from his legal marital obligations to provide her a home, economic support, and cohabitation. Neither could remarry, for that would be bigamy.

Though couples often favored separate maintenance agreements because of their extralegal standing, that standing could also become a disadvantage. The problem, at least for Jonathan, was that separate maintenance agreements had no legal teeth. Courts nearly always refused to enforce them, even when drafted by attorneys.[35] Jonathan had few options if Anna chose to disregard the terms on which they settled.[36]

And Anna chose to disregard the terms. She left neither Chillicothe nor the household, and she did not behave in a manner approved of by Jonathan. She did not change her behaviors to become the ideal doctor's wife. Leaving, it is important to point out, would have left her with no legal claim to her children. What she did do was take the money and make good financial investments. Within several years she had spent approximately one-third of the $3,000 by purchasing over nine hundred acres of land in Indiana, Illinois, and Wisconsin.[37] These land purchases, held in her name only, provided income until her death. Her actions, her refusal to go away, must have angered and frustrated Jonathan tremendously. While Anna's words are relayed only through Jonathan's legal narratives, her land purchases indicate agency, desire, and planning. She sought economic security independent from marriage and Jonathan. She sought to shape her own future.

In the spring of 1854, in the midst of marital discord and approximately a year after the failed separate maintenance agreement, Jonathan left town. Indeed, he left not only Chillicothe but also the United States from August 1854 to August 1855. When in 1859 he published a lengthy chronicle of his trip, he characterized the year as a religious pilgrimage, the result of "the ardent desire" of his heart "to stand upon the soil of Palestine where ancient Patriarchs lived and died, and the Son of Man himself taught, suffered and was crucified." He explained that "professional business" had previously kept him from such a trip but that "a favorable opportunity for one year's absence from home" had presented itself, and thus he embarked. Presumably, the "favorable opportunity" included a desire to escape his household. In reality, his pilgrimage to Egypt and Palestine lasted at maximum four months, and he appears to have spent the majority of his year in Paris.[38] He clearly had more than adequate financial resources: he had paid out $3,000 to Anna the year before and supported his Chillicothe household while traveling internationally for a year.

Meanwhile, Anna traveled to New York and boarded a ship for France.[39]

How many heretofore unknown wives, subsumed by historical presumptions of female and wifely unremarkableness into an archival void, engaged in similar efforts? Perhaps the lack of historical evidence signifies not a lack of action but a lack of the desire of others to recognize such action.

Esther, the hero of Charles Dickens's popular novel *Bleak House* (1852–53), characterized her life as a local doctor's wife as one of community adoration. Neighbors and townspeople, she said, adored her husband and adored her as an extension of him. "I never walk out with my husband but I hear the people bless him. I never go into a house of any degree but I hear his praises or see them in grateful eyes," the character raved. "The people even praise me as the doctor's wife. The people even like me as I go about, and make so much of me that I am quite abashed. I owe it all to him, my love, my pride! They like me for his sake, as I do everything I do in life for his sake."[40]

All remaining evidence, even that which points in contradictory directions, indicates that Anna Miesse's marriage and life in Chillicothe matched neither that of the fictional Esther nor that of marital guidebooks. Status, financial stability, and a legal marriage did not guarantee happiness for either husband or wife. The Miesse marriage, and all that the following few years would reveal, illustrates that amid the relatively forbidding strictures of mid-nineteenth-century marriage and property laws, and despite unpredictable consequences, husbands and wives, men and women, sought to shape their own lives.

2. The Questions of 1855

IN JUNE 1855 IN PARIS, the city of love, the couple reunited for the first time since Jonathan had left Chillicothe the previous August. As Jonathan described the scene, Anna "exaltingly acknowledged to him that she had kissed more than a hundred men since he had left home."[1] That teaser, however, is all that remains of the scene that Jonathan and Anna must have made somewhere in Paris. Perhaps Jonathan knew of Anna's arrival beforehand; perhaps she surprised him. After their reunion Anna remained in Europe. Jonathan began his return to the United States and in August arrived in Chillicothe to his medical practice, his children, and, undoubtedly, the rumors circulated by all his neighbors.

Nearly immediately upon his return, Jonathan retained an attorney and filed divorce papers again, after one withdrawn divorce attempt and one failed marital separation. Town gossip about the local doctor and his wife must have been rampant. Anna returned from Europe several months later. At this moment, her marital status and all that it legally, emotionally, and socially entailed left her limited options.

Before returning to Chillicothe for the early 1856 dismantling of the Miesse marriage, let us consider Anna's year while Jonathan traveled abroad. Jonathan's divorce complaint, Cornelius's school records, and various property documents chronicle the year. If Anna or an attorney retained by her testified in the divorce proceedings, the records do not remain. Virtually nothing of Anna's voice, even material created at her direction, remains in the historical record. Her May 1855 passport application is one exception. This source provides hints, perhaps loud intimations, that Anna B. Ott was complicated and messy. Dissonances between the various archival materials reverberate disconcertingly. Nineteenth-century white womanhood, even when buttressed by class and social status, was not monolithic. Nor was it always contained by the strictures and standards of respectable femininity.

When Jonathan left Chillicothe in August 1854 for Paris and Palestine he left sixteen-year-old Cornelius and seven-year-old Aurelia in the care of their mother and household servants. Per Jonathan's 1855 divorce complaint, while he was gone for the year Anna "drove" Cornelius away from home with such "harsh treatment" that the young man sought refuge with a nearby relative. Moving to a relative's home is plausible, particularly considering that Jonathan's many brothers and their households resided in Ohio, as did Anna's parents and nearly all of her twelve siblings. Turning seventeen in December 1854, Cornelius was old enough to undertake such a move on his own. Unmentioned in Jonathan's complaint, however, is Cornelius's enrollment at Ohio Wesleyan University (Delaware, Ohio) during the 1854–55 academic year. Cornelius was away at school. While he perhaps returned home at times during school sessions, the seventy-two miles between Chillicothe and Delaware were not an easy trip. Anna's "harsh treatment" did not drive him to leave home during the school year, classes did, as they had the prior academic year.[2] Jonathan misled the court.

Anna left Chillicothe multiple times during the year of her husband's absence. Jonathan's divorce complaint states that approximately two months after his departure Anna "remained absent from her family" for six weeks, "leaving her son and daughter in the charge of servants, and otherwise neglecting" the two children. The reality was that Cornelius remained at boarding school, and perhaps Aurelia did also. Jonathan's divorce complaint states that prior to his fall 1854 departure he placed Aurelia in school, "to remain until his return home."[3] Legally, these decisions were his alone to make. Chillicothe hosted the Chillicothe Female Seminary, a respectable private school for young white girls. Aurelia likely boarded at the school, as other girls of the Chillicothe elite did. "Neglect" was an exaggeration if not an outright misrepresentation, though Anna did travel. Between October and January she purchased land in Illinois, Indiana, and Wisconsin, probably using the money she had received from Jonathan in the 1853 marital separation agreement. She likely inspected possible land purchases during those months and worked with land agents in each region. Anna then traveled farther from home, perhaps for the first time since her 1834 immigration to the United States. In May she applied for a passport while in New York. In June she and her husband argued in Paris.

Anna's May 1855 passport application provides the first physical description of her that remains, one of only two descriptions. She had "a dark complexion," accompanied by "auburn hair, hazel eyes, good teeth, square shoulders," and she was "strongly built with a height of five feet three inches and three quarters of an inch."[4]

A passport application required that someone else attest to the individual's identity and truthfulness. Jacob S. Atwood, a prominent Chillicothe banker who at that time worked on New York's Wall Street and who had built a prominent Chillicothe home the same year that Jonathan and Anna did, swore to the notary that "the said Anna B. Miesse is a person of good moral character and has been to him known as such for sixteen years last past." Other than Atwood's presence in New York, why he did this or why Anna turned to him is unknown. While just over a year later Jonathan would make claims about his wife's scandalous behavior and her local notoriety, at the time of the passport application Atwood testified to the "good moral character" of the local doctor's wife.[5]

Most striking are the additional biographical facts sworn to in Mrs. Anna Miesse's passport application. Anna, the notarized document attested, was "a graduate of the Female Medical College of Philadelphia, a practitioner of medicine, and a physician for at least three years." The notary public attested that Anna had proven her profession via "diplomatic evidence," that is, with supporting paperwork.[6]

Did Anna B. Miesse graduate from medical school? Had she served as a physician for at least three years prior to 1855? Did she produce a medical school diploma for the New York notary?

None of these things is impossible.

Anna, married to Jonathan since 1837, undoubtedly knew that female physicians existed. Whether or not Jonathan and his brothers supported the controversial entrance of women into medical schools, they likely discussed the issue at their professional meetings, perhaps conversed about it at their dining-room tables, and read of it in newspapers and medical journals. Jonathan presumably encountered supporters of female physicians or even a female physician herself, particularly during his years in Philadelphia.

Women fought to attend medical school and be taken seriously as medical professionals in the mid-nineteenth century. The number of women who attended medical school was very small, but they and other women who sought to do so garnered significant attention. Elizabeth Blackwell began at Geneva Medical College (New York) in 1847, though the school admitted no other women at the time. Boston hosted the New England Female Medical College beginning in 1848. And while Jonathan's alma mater did not admit women, two Philadelphia institutions did: the Female Medical College of Pennsylvania began to do so in 1850, and Penn Medical University accepted them in 1851. Neither, however, admitted women between 1844 and 1846, the years Jonathan spent in Philadelphia. In 1850 the Cleveland Homeopathic College opened its doors to both men and women. Even closer to home, in multiple ways, was the Eclectic Medical College of Cincinnati, which Jonathan's brother Gabriel had attended during the 1846–47 school year. Cincinnati was just over one hundred miles away, and the Eclectic Medical College had allowed a female to attend only two years after Gabriel.[7]

It is, however, improbable that Anna attended medical school.

Despite my best historical mining efforts, I have found no documentation of Anna Barbara Blaser Miesse (or Ott) in the records of any of the possible medical schools in Philadelphia, Ohio, New York, or elsewhere. Even more so, the timing does not work. No Philadelphia schools accepted women during the years Jonathan attended medical school in Philadelphia, and thus Anna did not attend medical school while he did. The years when schools accepting women were open do not correspond to Anna's life of marriage and childbearing and to her husband's education. Though I want Anna to have gone to medical school, my belief is that in her 1855 passport application Anna B. Miesse simply lied about having gone to medical school.

It is highly likely, however, that Anna had medical expertise—indeed, far more than some male physicians. The nearly twenty years of Anna's marriage to Jonathan, whose house served as a primary medical workspace, constituted a lengthy apprenticeship. Indeed, Jonathan's initial apprenticeship had likely lasted only several months. Jonathan had gone to medical school, but only after ten years of already practicing; and most men recognized as physicians never went to school. Medical school was not a requirement for serving and being publicly recognized as a doctor. In the domestic sphere of the Miesse home and as a local doctor's wife, Anna would have helped with surgeries and other procedures, manufactured and cleaned medical equipment, welcomed patients while Jonathan was absent and performed necessary triage, received messages requesting Jonathan's assistance, overheard hours of medical conversation, and had ready access to his medical books and supplies. In other words, she knew mid-nineteenth-century medicine, and she likely knew it well.

Why Anna bothered to get a passport and why she claimed having gone to medical school are unclear. Neither was necessary. The United States and European nations did not require passports at their borders at this time.[8] Perhaps it was due to ease of travel. Anna may have believed that fellow travelers would find a married woman en route to join her husband more socially acceptable than a single woman traveling alone. She may have hoped that a professional and educated woman embodied respectability. A passport testified that she was who she said she was, even with a passport's only vaguely official and legal standing in 1855.

And beyond that, why go to Europe?

It is tempting to speculate, but such speculation is my own desire to render tidy an archival void and to assemble Anna in ways that appeal to my contemporary tastes. I want her to have gone to Europe to sneak in a medical education, to have carried out undocumented family business on behalf of her parents, to have had a passionate love affair, or to have chased down treasures in Paris.

While this period and its scant evidence raise nearly unlimited questions with unknown answers, abundantly clear are the economic and racial privileges of the Miesse household. Whether male or female, husband or wife, Jonathan and Anna both had personal, legal, and economic resources on which to draw.

3. *Miesse v. Miesse*, 1856

LIKE ALL MEN AND WOMEN who entered into legal marriage in the mid-nineteenth-century United States, when Jonathan and Anna said their marital vows in 1837 they entered into a legal contract that committed both individuals to significant obligations in pursuit of marital unity. Anna's duties within the marital contract were to give Jonathan complete access to her property and labor—her physical goods, household labor, wages, sex, physical presence, and the bearing and raising of children. He had "possessory right" over her body and production. Unless Anna had property that was legally specified as a separate estate, she had no personal possessions—everything was Jonathan's. Jonathan had a duty to provide Anna with goods and a domicile.

When Dr. Jonathan Miesse petitioned the court to dissolve his marital contract after returning from a year of international travel, he did so within a very specific and very limited legal framework. A divorce petition could come from only one spouse, and for the marital contract to be rendered null, the other spouse had to be determined guilty of wrongdoing. Divorce could not happen unless one spouse took the blame. Divorce "required guilt, and it required innocence, and it required a public decision and clear proof that one spouse and one spouse only, had fundamentally breached his or her obligations as a spouse."[1] No evidence indicates that Anna sought to have a divorce complaint issued against Jonathan (though Ohio wives could and did). If Jonathan wanted a divorce, he had to prove that Anna had engaged in impotency, bigamy, adultery, desertion, habitual drunkenness, fraudulent contract, imprisonment, or a "total of gross neglect of duty."[2] If Anna agreed to a divorce initiated by Jonathan, she had to be guilty, or agree to be found guilty, of one or more items on this list. An easier strategy, and one far more likely to be adopted by individuals with few economic resources, was to simply desert the relationship and remake oneself under a new name in a new place.

With the aid of an attorney, Jonathan Miesse (the complainant) thus submitted a divorce complaint against Anna B. Miesse (the defendant) on September 4, 1855. Because he was dependent on his medical practice and medical degree and was imbedded in a network of extended family members, desertion would not have been a favorable option for him. He must have been frustrated, for he had already withdrawn one divorce complaint, and the separate maintenance agreement had failed. Anna remained away from Chillicothe (in Switzerland at the time, according to Jonathan's legal filings), and thus the court issued a summons for her to appear before it in early November. By late November she had hired an attorney (presumably with money she had gained in the 1853 attempted separation). Per her attorney's request, the court ordered Jonathan to continue his obligations of support: each month he was to provide fifty dollars "to furnish the said Anna B. Miesse with provisions, fuel and servants suitable, and sufficient for herself and child [presumably Aurelia] at the residence of the petitioner." In other words, Anna remained in their Chillicothe home with Aurelia. Where Jonathan lived is unstated.[3]

The divorce complaint drawn by Jonathan's legal counsel began by establishing the legitimacy of their marriage and children, and it acknowledged the withdrawn 1849 divorce petition. Jonathan, the complaint summarized, had always fulfilled his parts of the marital contract with "uniform kindness," while Anna was "turbulent, quarrelsome, and grossly neglectful of her duty" to Jonathan and their children. Gross neglect of duty remained vital to the divorce's legal success. A week before the judge issued his ruling, in March 1856, Jonathan's attorney submitted a second litany of complaints. Including the entirety of the two complaints, Anna's alleged wrongs were quite substantial.[4] The accusations against Anna fall into four general but overlapping categories: she defamed Jonathan's personal character, she damaged his professional livelihood, she neglected their children and household, and she engaged in adultery and other inappropriate gender/sexual behaviors. In all ways, he claimed she neglected her duties as his wife.[5] Such accusations fulfilled two of Ohio's then criteria for divorce: gross neglect of duty and adultery.

Anna allegedly defamed her husband's personal character in multiple ways. She accused him of lewd behavior with lewd women. She "capriciously" refused to cooperate in real estate management, "thereby putting him to much trouble and inconvenience." It seemed to particularly infuriate Jonathan that he arrived home from his year abroad to find that she had "falsely informed sundry persons" to whom he owed debts that he would never return, resulting in lawsuits "to the infamy of his name and credit." Compounding the alleged damage to Jonathan's personal character was alleged damage to his professional standing. The complaint stated that Anna had accused Jonathan and his medical partners of being mediocre physicians and charged at least one partner of sexual relations with "lewd" women. Jonathan claimed she "intervened, insulted, charged with stealing, and abused and in several instances has violently assaulted or beaten" his medical partners and apprentices. She harassed his patients, using "abusive, profane, and obscure language towards male and female patients." She stole medical books, medical equipment, and mail related to the medical practice.[6]

Jonathan also charged Anna with "gross neglect of duty, and extreme cruelty, both towards complainant and his children." She insulted him in front of their children, used "profane and vulgar language before both of her children," never had meals ready, and had attacked him "as many as ten or twelve times, with a club, or other convenient weapons and forced him from fear of bodily harm to fly from the house." Several of these attacks Jonathan detailed at length.[7] She had tried to cause the poisoning of "a much respected friend." On "ten or fifteen occasions she has violently assaulted and beaten and threatened her son Cornelius in various modes," and she accused both her husband and son of "adultery, fornication, theft, perjury, attempts at rape, and other such crimes." Jonathan and Cornelius, the petition claimed, lived "constantly in fear of bodily injury, or of loss of life, from her." In addition, during Jonathan's yearlong absence she had "neglected" the two children during her travels and had left them with no financial resources.[8] Other than references to "the children," the divorce complaint said very little about Aurelia.

Finally, Jonathan accused Anna of a long list of sexual and gender transgressions that met the adultery criteria of Ohio divorce law. Specifically, Jonathan charged Anna with "the crime of adultery with one Lewis Allen," "a man of notoriously licentious character," as well as "diverse other lewd men." Jonathan claimed that during his yearlong absence, Anna had, "regardless of her duty and example before her children," "kept the company of said Allen, in the presence of her said children, within her own house, on numberless occasions . . . and after remained alone with him to late hours of the night." This created a "scandal," Jonathan claimed, and despite "the complaint made to her by her friends and neighbors in relation thereof, she refused to dismiss said Allen from her house." In the company of the household's hired man she used "profane and lascivious speech" and wore clothing of an "obscene manner." While she had traveled to purchase land "she frequently consorted and kept company with men of licentious habits" and continued in correspondence with at least one of those licentious men.[9]

More broadly, Anna allegedly behaved "in a manner incompatible with the character of a chaste and virtuous wife [and] mother." Jonathan's divorce complaint charged that she frequently left the house "late in the afternoon or early in the evening, unaccompanied by any one, and remaining away until midnight or thereabouts." She had, he claimed, "demeaned herself with gross familiarity and impropriety in the presence of *sundry persons of both sexes*." Furthermore, she had been seen frequently visiting a local "house of known doubtful repute for chastity"—a brothel—and "on diverse occasions appreciated *with men and other persons*" under circumstances that created "strong and just suspicions." In addition, she had cross-dressed: on "one or more occasions" she dressed "her person in male attire at night." Despite the lengthy list, Jonathan's attorney wrote that Anna's specified wrongs were "only a part of an immeasurable number of acts of similar nature."[10] Jonathan's word was his evidence. He provided no other substantiation. If all or even most of these allegations were true, Anna was neither the typical nor the desired wife of any mid-nineteenth-century Ohio physician.

Before the judge issued his final decision on the Miesse divorce Jonathan withdrew the charge of adultery. The case records provide no explanation. Perhaps Anna objected particularly strenuously to this part of the complaint; perhaps she agreed to not object to "gross neglect" if Jonathan dropped the adultery charges. Perhaps the charges weren't true. Perhaps attorneys advised Jonathan that the allegations lacked adequate proof, and thus the divorce would not be granted on these terms. Perhaps Jonathan did not want to be thought of as a cuckold. As historian Thomas Buckley has written, "At its center adultery by women defied male domination. If in any sense these cuckolds might be called patriarchs, at best they were deviant ones."[11]

Whatever the reason, on March 15, 1856, the Honorable John L. Green, judge of the Court of Common Pleas for the County, found Anna B. Miesse "guilty of the gross neglect of duty." Anna bore the legal wrong of neglecting her marital duties and thus was determined to be the guilty party in the divorce. The judge dissolved the marital contract and declared both to be "wholly released from the obligations therewith."[12] Jonathan Miesse and Anna Miesse were now divorced. Cornelius was eighteen, Aurelia nine.

This divorce case, including accusations of late-night cross-dressing adventures and brothel visits, as well as innuendos of sexual relationships, undoubtedly stood out as unique among Ohio cases.

Discerning the truth of Jonathan's allegations is complex. He and his attorney laid out a remarkable and long barrage of Anna's legal, moral, and gender transgressions. Doth Jonathan protest too much? Turning to others may help unpack his allegations. Pulling out Anna's voice, actions, and experience of marriage from the content of Jonathan Miesse's divorce complaint, however, is difficult. The voices of their children, Cornelius and Aurelia, are not present. Jonathan's colleagues or patients, purportedly attacked, did not testify in the divorce proceedings. Extended family members and neighbors don't appear in these records, which is unusual. The only other individual present in the legal records was Judge Green.

Judge John Green's 1856 analysis of the Miesse marriage and the behaviors of both husband and wife is revealed in his final judgment and in the details of the financial and child custody settlements he crafted. Green determined Anna guilty of gross neglect, but his findings were far more subtle than a simple determination of Jonathan as innocent and Anna as guilty.

Anna stepped away from the Miesse marriage a wealthy woman. Though she lost all future dower rights (access to one-third of Jonathan's estate for the purpose of supporting herself after his death) and all future claims to Jonathan's financial support, Judge Green settled upon her significant financial gains. Arguably, the result was *better* than a dower right, in which case she would not have had control of the funds and could not have determined where they went after she died. Anna kept all results of the $3,000 Jonathan had given her in March 1853: the over nine hundred acres of land, the $939.50 in a local bank, and all that came from an investment earning 10 percent annual interest. In addition, the judge required Jonathan to pay the legal expenses of both of them and to pay Anna an additional $1,000 over each of the next three years ($3,000 beyond the $3,000 already given her in 1853). She was to own all "as her own separate property."[13] For comparison, $3,000 in 1855 equaled approximately $100,533 in 2018.[14] Neither Jonathan nor any future husband would have claim to her property.

Anna also stepped away from the Miesse marriage with considerable access to Aurelia, particularly considering that child custody usually "went readily to the allegedly innocent spouse."[15] Jonathan received "custody" of the eighteen-year-old college-attending Cornelius. Nine-year-old Aurelia was to live with Anna, but Jonathan retained the right to "remove her" if he ever "render[ed] such removal necessary or proper." Jonathan retained control of decisions regarding Aurelia's education but in exchange had to contribute seventy-five dollars to her education each year.[16]

All in all, other than laying the legal wrongs on Anna, Judge John Green did not punish her. Purportedly, Anna exercised great violence, attacking Jonathan with a knife, a fire poker, and a broom handle, only thwarted when restrained by others. Yet though the divorce petition claimed that Jonathan and Cornelius were "constantly in fear of bodily injury, or of loss of life" due to Anna's threats and actions, the judge *and* Jonathan allowed Aurelia to live with her mother. This suggests that the claims of Anna's violence were either false or exaggerated. And if Anna's sexual activities were those that Jonathan's divorce petition maintained, it is unlikely that either the judge or Jonathan would have so willingly agreed to Aurelia living with her mother. The fact that Aurelia stayed with Anna strongly suggests that the judge, the general community, and perhaps even Jonathan did not embrace the complete veracity of Jonathan's accusations.

Had Jonathan and Anna colluded to lie in order to be divorced?

Perhaps it is useful to consider what was *not* included in Jonathan's divorce complaint. Jonathan made no attempt to sue any of Anna's alleged adultery partners, even the specific Lewis Allen, for "theft of affection." He did not file a civil action for "criminal conversation" to recover damages from his wife's seducer. Perhaps Jonathan didn't care. Perhaps the allegations were untrue or unprovable. Either strategy placed legal blame on an alleged male partner, not on Anna, and did not give Jonathan a divorce. Either strategy removed the *action*, the *agency* of the wrong from Anna. Both strategies instead remedied "the wrongs that men did to each other" rather than the wrong Anna did to Jonathan.[17] Divorce required proof of legal wrong, and Jonathan wanted the legal wrong to fall on Anna.

The evidence suggests collusion and suggests that all, including Judge Green, knew so. Because nineteenth-century divorces required either husband or wife to be guilty of very specific legal wrongs, some couples colluded in order to obtain a divorce. In such cases, evidence had to be manufactured, staged, or stretched so that one party could be determined guilty of wrongdoings worthy of divorce. Dissatisfaction and unhappiness were not enough. Despite prohibitions against collusion, colonial and then state courts had long known of it, sometimes berating, sometimes tolerating the practice. In regions with "clear and limited grounds for divorce" collusions existed. Indeed, as historian Hendrik Hartog has written, "Perjury, collusion, fiction were all crucial parts of divorce practice."[18] Historian David Silkenat found evidence that in nineteenth-century North Carolina couples in agreement about ending a marriage sometimes "arranged for only one of them to file for divorce" in order to speed and ease the process.[19]

The possibility of collusion forces a rereading of the divorce allegations. For example, Jonathan charged that while Anna had traveled to purchase land "she frequently consorted and kept company with men of licentious habits" and then continued in correspondence with such men.[20] Perhaps she had enjoyed the company of other men. It is also possible, however, that she worked and then corresponded with male land agents, a common practice in this period when women's property laws varied from state to state and when sellers could refuse to sell to women.

Reading some of Jonathan's divorce petition allegations while considering Anna's extensive medical knowledge and her later twenty-year medical career additionally problematizes the allegations. Anna allegedly stole much of Jonathan's medical equipment. She reputedly went out at night, sometimes in men's clothing, and was "seen frequently to visit a house of known doubtful repute for chastity in the city of Chillicothe." She purportedly "demeaned herself with gross familiarity and impropriety in the presence of sundry persons of both sexes—in a manner incompatible with the character of a chaste and virtuous wife mother."[21] Later divorce suits that involved Anna included a pile of impressive allegations but never included allegations of sexual impropriety.

Many female physicians in this period faced charges of sexual impropriety simply because their medical practice included exposure to the bodies of male and female patients in various states of undress. A physical exam or medical treatment generally required a patient to remove at least some of his or her clothing. Anna could have been practicing medicine at night, sometimes visiting brothels to do so, and in the process would have had intimate exposure to men's and women's bodies. Chillicothe had no lack of poor people or brothels. Anna had access to medical equipment, and she had medical knowledge. She would later practice medicine for twenty years. If Anna had been poaching on the medical turf of Chillicothe's male medical practitioners, and if her patients paid her, she surely would have incurred the wrath of Jonathan and other local physicians straining for respectability. Anna's engagement in such activities could have made collusion more acceptable to members of the community who supported this specific divorce.

Historical readings of nineteenth-century divorce cases in this period provide ample evidence that "divorce petitioners carefully crafted their legal filings" in a predictable narrative that firmly established the guilt of one party and the innocence of another. The narrative strategies of men seeking divorce began by establishing their long forbearance and patience, contrasted "their wives' behavior with an ideal of feminine temperament and behavior," and concluded by emphasizing "their wives' sexual depravity, often charging them with prostitution."[22] Jonathan's successful divorce petition exemplifies this legal and narrative formula. The petition carefully emphasized Anna's gross neglect. Jonathan began with the claim that he had always fulfilled "the duties of a provident, liberal, faithful, and affectionate husband," noted that he had chosen to unhappily "bear with her frailties than suffer the mortification of an open rupture with her," and then insisted that his wife's transgressions had become too horrendous to endure. She had become "without cause or provocation . . . turbulent, quarrelsome, and grossly neglectful of her duty" toward her husband and children.[23] As in so many cases in which a male divorce petitioner alleged his wife's adultery, Jonathan presented the adultery "as a repudiation of an idyllic union."[24]

Silkenat argues that, at least in North Carolina, the number of divorce petitioners who chose "this particular narrative mode" suggests that "it must have been a successful strategy both in persuading the judge and jury to grant the divorce and in mitigating the disgrace of divorce"—the disgrace, at least, for Jonathan.[25] Within eight months of the divorce he married a woman sixteen years his junior and five years older than his son, Cornelius. His new bride, Elizabeth "Eliza" Kennedy, moved into the house over which Anna had presided for thirteen years and became the local doctor's wife. He continued to live and practice his career in Chillicothe until his death many decades later. The divorce and its spectacular charges appear to have had little impact on his long-term financial and social standing.

Someone had to be guilty for Anna and Jonathan to divorce. The formulaic narrative of Jonathan's divorce petition, the monetary and child custody award given to Anna, and the dramatically sensationalistic nature of his allegations suggest that not all the statements were true. Marriage and patriarchy, however, created a legal context in which Anna and Jonathan faced limited options. If she sought to end the marriage, she may have had to accept marital guilt in order to gain Jonathan's acquiescence. If he determinedly sought to end the marriage, she would have been wise to accept marital guilt in exchange for financial resources. In March 1856 the Chillicothe, Ohio, court determined Anna and Jonathan's marriage to be over. The stigma and shame of divorce landed resolutely on Anna. Silkenat found that more than 95 percent of divorced people between 1830 and 1860 left town for a new life, and Anna did the same.[26]

Whatever truths lay or did not lie within Jonathan's divorce petitions, it is clear that charges of sexual and gender behaviors inappropriate for a woman of her class and marital status rendered Mrs. Anna B. Miesse socially illegitimate. They had impact and power. For Jonathan and other husbands like him, accusations of sexual infamy and unwomanliness served as effective strategies either to restrain a wife's undesirable behaviors or to get rid of her. Anna lost her wifely status and became a divorced woman. Given the later pathologization of Anna's behaviors and the immense consequences of such ableist pathologization, it is notable that these tumultuous marital proceedings included no accusations of insanity.

Despite the relatively strict and formal legal boundaries of mid-nineteenth-century marriage law, however, this is not an example of overwhelming victimhood. In a decade in which early women's rights activists were only beginning to prod state legislators to pass laws enabling women to own and control their own property and in which many divorced women lost access to their children, Mrs. Anna Miesse emerged from the marriage with access to her daughter, Aurelia, and at least $6,000. This was a moment at which much could happen.

4. The Questions of 1856

IMMEDIATELY AFTER THE DIVORCE, Anna's life entered a period for which little documentation exists. Once again, the historical figure does not listen to her biographer, who wishes her to do something momentous and leave behind remaining evidence. Instead, what she did and where she went after the Chillicothe court finalized her 1856 divorce from Jonathan Miesse are unclear. It is possible and likely that the thirty-six-year-old Anna returned to the home of her parents near Winesburg, Ohio. Both parents were still alive, and several of her large number of siblings lived nearby.

Where Anna's youngest sister, Sophia, lived throughout much of the 1850s also is unclear and matters to what happened next. Before 1850 the unmarried Sophia had moved into the Miesse household in Chillicothe, likely to help with the children and household tasks. Living with a married sister gave her respectability and something to do while escaping the watchfulness of her parents. Sometime in this period Sophia met George V. Ott, a recent German immigrant who had settled in Richland County, Ohio. She and George married in 1852, before her twenty-first birthday, and she bore their only child, George F. S. Ott, sometime in 1853. In 1855 Sophia died. Why, where, and exactly when she died are lost to the historical record.[1]

George and Sophia matter to this story because Anna married her sister's widower just a few months after the divorce from Jonathan. How Sophia died may matter to this story because of Anna's later allegations of George's violence.

George can be characterized as a slippery character, but perhaps that is unfair, for he is no more slippery than most nonfamous nineteenth-century individuals. The records are simply hard to find, for both George and Ott were common names. White male biographical subjects, however, tended to be kind to their biographers and maintain the same name throughout their lives in this period. This George Ott was one of the many men and women who left Germany in the aftermath and confusion of the 1848 Revolution. He settled first in Shelby, Ohio, and worked in a tannery owned by other German immigrants. He married and buried Sophia. Two of his brothers joined him in 1855, but in 1856 he left them and moved to Madison, Wisconsin. His two brothers remained in Shelby for the rest of their lives. In Madison, George established what would become a successful tannery, manufacturing and selling various leather goods.

George married his dead wife's oldest sister, Anna, a woman about seven years his senior (an unusual age gap), in the spring of 1856.[2] It is easy to dismiss Anna and George's marriage as too soon after the divorce or Sophia's death. The marriage, which took place at the Holmes County Lutheran church, which Anna and Sophia's father had helped to found (perhaps even the church in which Anna and Jonathan had married and in which Sophia and George had married), occurred approximately two months after the divorce and, at most, just over a year after Sophia's death. I do not know when Anna and George started their relationship. I do not know what the extended Blaser family thought of the marriage. Nor do I know what Anna's children, Cornelius and Aurelia, thought. Anna and George went on to raise his son, George F. S. Ott, who was Anna's young nephew and her children's cousin. Perhaps the marriage was simply convenient and practical. George was a widower, Anna was divorced, and someone needed to raise the young George. A marriage bestowed respectability on Anna. By the fall, George, Anna, Aurelia, and the young George (six years younger than Aurelia) lived in Madison, Wisconsin. The exact chronology of Sophia's death, Anna's purchase of land in Wisconsin, George and Anna's relationship, Jonathan and Eliza's relationship, and the departure of George and Anna for Madison matters but can only be pinned down to the inexact period of 1855 and 1856.

An additional unanswered question is the nature of George and Sophia's marriage. This matters not just for the sake of a good story or to add to titillating speculations about George and Anna's relationship. The nature of George and Sophia's marriage matters because the marriage of George and Anna quickly became turbulent, with evidence of significant violence. I do not know if George and Sophia's marriage included violence, but George and Anna's certainly did, and it is unlikely that George was violent in one relationship and not in another. If George and Sophia's marriage had been violent, perhaps Anna had known of it, for Sophia had lived in the Miesse household. If Anna did know of the violence between her sister and George, that leaves the frustrating question of why Anna married George when she had no economic necessity to do so.

Then there are questions regarding George and his progeny. At the time of George and Anna's wedding, George had a three-year-old son, who had been birthed by Sophia (George F. S. Ott). George also had a second son, birthed by another man's wife at an unspecified time; the son and woman are mentioned briefly but not named in a much later court case. One wonders if either Sophia or Anna knew of this son and this relationship. Where the woman lived and when she gave birth to George's son is a mystery. The lack of names, locations, and dates provides no evidence with which to pursue them.

An additional question regards a young girl named Minetta Monona Ott, born March 7, 1856, in Madison—the day before Jonathan withdrew the adultery charge against Anna, eight days before the legal declaration of the Miesse divorce, and approximately two months before George and Anna married.[3] Minetta's parentage is confusing. Historical records regarding Minetta consistently name George as her father but only occasionally reference a mother and name Anna when doing so. Where she grew up is unclear. There is no reference to her in the 1860 census; the 1870 census lists George and Anna as her parents but indicates her to be away "at school." As an adult Minetta listed her father as having been born in Germany (as George had been) and her mother in Switzerland (as Anna had been).

It is possible but not likely that Anna gave birth to Minetta, fathered by George, in March 1856. Anna had traveled to Wisconsin to purchase land, and it is conceivable that she had then given birth to a child, whom she left in someone's care and to whom she returned that fall when the new Mr. and Mrs. Ott moved to Madison. However, if Minetta was full term and born on March 7, that means that she was conceived in early June 1855. Though Anna traveled the Midwest purchasing land during 1855, in early June she was in Paris confronting Jonathan and could not have conceived a child with George. And if Anna had been pregnant in early 1856, surely Jonathan would have included that fact in the divorce allegations. An 1881 court case states that George and Anna never had children. George and Anna's tumultuous marriage entered court documents many times, but the records never mentioned Minetta. It is likely that Anna did not give birth to Minetta.

The questions only compound, however, if George fathered Minetta with another woman. One wonders what happened to the woman and why Anna would agree to raise a young girl, apparently a daughter of George's, born just months before her marriage to George. Even more perplexing is why Anna would agree to marry George if he already had two children outside of his marriage to her sister. Regardless of unanswered questions, Minetta came from somewhere and then lived as George and Anna's daughter, at least for a while. Whatever the details, this was not the marital and sexual blandness of nineteenth-century historical mythology.

Though the legal strictures of marriage and wifehood changed little between Anna's first marriage in 1837 and her second in 1856, the acquisition of financial resources in her own name and the lessons she had learned as a local doctor's wife dramatically altered Anna's social and legal standing. The forces propelling her internally are nearly impossible to discern; were they boredom, a desire for money, love of her children, a desire to escape patriarchy and exercise her own agency, the struggle of a psychiatric disability, or simple desperation and loneliness? Discernable, however, are the historical forces acting upon her and in which she maneuvered. Marital and property laws, the patriarchal social structures they upheld, along with privileges of class and profession had a tremendous impact upon the life of the woman born Anna Barbara Blaser.

This chapter is a list of questions based on an inexact and frustratingly limited historical record. At the core of this confusing chronology and array of questions are the sparse facts that Sophia died, Jonathan and Anna divorced, and George and Anna married. This would be a different book if one or several of the involved individuals had kept a detailed calendar of the events of 1855 and 1856 and left it for me to find, along with letters or a diary containing juicy personal secrets. Family members who labored hard to keep their knowledge of the events away from neighbors may have strengthened the void, as did the later isolation of Anna from her extended family.

This archival void, like many archival voids, is not simply random or due only to family scandals. It is no accident that it is easier to write the biography of an individual who has power and high status. In this case, as in many cases, the lack of historical records indicates the existence of devalued human beings rather than the lack of human beings. Supposed unimportance due to race, class, gender, or ability resulted in limited evidentiary trails and archival omission. Marriage and property laws, for example, often wrote white women and all those peoples legally barred from accessing marriage or property out of the archives. The resulting archival voids make biography difficult and directly determine which biographies historians construct and which they do not. It is vital that historians consider these methodological dilemmas; otherwise, we, via our craft itself, either replicate the power structures of the past or present them as natural and inevitable.

5. Dr. Anna B. Ott, Local Doctress

IN 1856, BY ESTABLISHING herself as a professional physician, marrying her widowed brother-in-law, George Ott, and then moving to Madison, Wisconsin, the newly renamed Mrs. Dr. Anna B. Ott transformed herself. Instead of a local doctor's wife, instead of an impugned divorcee, Anna became a doctor and property owner. Privileges of money, whiteness, marital status, the claim to a profession, and the relative distance between the new state of Wisconsin and the more established settler regions that hosted medical schools accepting female students facilitated the transformation. Though patriarchy and sexism meant that female physicians often encountered resistance and outright hostility in the mid-nineteenth century, Dr. Anna B. Ott declared herself a graduate of a medical college and opened her practice. Being a doctor was more powerful than being a doctor's wife. Arriving as a married female physician who had graduated from a medical college was less dubious than arriving single.

The mid-nineteenth century held potential for geographic and personal remaking, particularly for whites able to garner adequate financial resources. This "new world of strangers" offered spaces in which inhabitants could verify little of the personal histories of their neighbors and community members. From 1820 to 1860 the population of the United States grew by 226 percent, while the proportion of people living in cities grew 797 percent.[1] From 1850 to 1860, immediately after Wisconsin statehood in 1848, the population of the city of Madison grew by 395 percent.[2] In this world of strangers, no one would question the motives and histories of individual new arrivals amid the large waves of people.

The newly married Anna and George Ott settled in Madison in the fall of 1856, along with nine-year-old Aurelia, four-year-old George, and perhaps the infant Minetta. Why they picked Madison is a mystery, but the economy of the region and its white settler population were growing quickly, and no one there knew or knew of them. In 1848 Congress declared the Ho Chunk tribal territory a US state. In May 1854 the first railroad arrived in Madison to an eager and excited crowd of over two thousand people. In the spring of 1855 a local newspaper reported, "Never before was the building mania in Madison more apparent than now. . . . It seems that everybody is coming to Madison." In 1856 the city's first opera house opened, and in 1857 the state legislature approved funds for a new state capitol.[3] Despite panic about the Dakota Uprising of 1862 across the border in Minnesota, white settlers remained in control of the region. These white settlers became Anna Ott's paying patients. For someone with money, such as Anna, the growing city offered significant investment opportunities. She bought more land, including several business properties on the square that surrounded the site of the state capitol.

Feminist activists, a few protective fathers, and a variety of social reformers contested marital norms and the rights of husbands to their wives' bodies, property, and earnings in this period. Loosening divorce laws were part of the process by which "the companionate ideal [of marriage] became imbedded in law" and by which Anna and Jonathan had divorced.[4] The wave of women's property laws that swept through the last half of the nineteenth century granted women greater control of their property, even within marriage. Male household violence became "less acceptable" than in earlier decades.[5] Marital violence in Wisconsin, however, was "elevated and ferocious" compared to regions in which settler colonialism was more firmly established. Historian Robin Sager argues, "Wisconsin society in the 1840s and 1850s was still a frontier. . . . [I]t appears as if Wisconsin men took their cues from the violence that they witnessed in their communities and perpetrated physical marital cruelties as part of a quest to reinforce their authority as the head of a household."[6] This suggests that the normalized violence committed by settler colonialists against indigenous communities leaked into settler households and relationships. This is another example of how, in addition to the creation of courts and governing institutions such as the Wisconsin State Hospital for the Insane, settler colonialism shaped the lives of Wisconsin settlers.

In this context Anna married George, a man who, perhaps, had already had one violent marriage. George opened a tannery and leather goods business in one of Anna's storefronts on Pinckney Street, eventually selling harnesses and shoes and employing as many as twenty people. George thus paid rent to his wife for the use of both the lot and the building in what must have been a rare marital arrangement.[7] Violence and ableism would permeate the rest of Anna's life as an individual and then as one member of a large institutionalized population. Individual privileges and violent patriarchy blended in confusing ways in this period of Anna's life. The medical profession provided her with status and resources, misogynistic hostility, a stigmatized diagnosis, and eventual incarceration in this period.

Over 1858 and 1859 the couple employed the local architectural firm of Donnell and Kutzboch to build a grand home, one of many ornate brick or sandstone homes built in this decade in the growing town. The architectural duo also designed the state capitol, authorized in 1857, and by hiring them, George and Anna made clear their desire to be part of the Madison elite. What later became known as the Ott-Wright home was situated at 21 East Wilson Street, facing the capitol and downtown and along the shore of Lake Monona. Originally, an iron fence surrounded the brick home, two porches sat on both sides of the front door, a driveway ran along the right side, and a barn lay between the house and the lake.[8] Students of architecture would later note an "eccentric feature" of the house: every room, including the wine cellar and attic, had both an entrance and an exit door.[9] Aurelia lived with them, as did Anna's nephew and George's son, George F. S. Ott, and, perhaps, Minetta.[10]

While George opened a tannery and leather goods business, Anna established herself as a physician—or, as the 1866 Madison city directory listed her, a "medical doctress."[11] Discerning the extent of Anna's medical practice is difficult, for no records remain. At various points in these decades both she and George repeated the claim that she had graduated from medical school, and no one seems to have challenged that claim. Though she frequently was not listed among physicians in the city directories, sometimes she was. Newspaper articles, legal records, the couple's financial records, the records of Anna's institutionalization, and at least one medical association recognized her as a physician in dates that range from 1857 to immediately after her death in 1893. One legal record indicated her financial gains from her profession as substantial.[12] While not embraced by area male medical professionals, she was recognized as such and in some cases was called "Mrs. Dr. Ott."

In the late 1850s only one "other" female medical college graduate lived in Wisconsin. Dr. Laura J. Ross Wollcott began a practice in Milwaukee after graduating from the Women's Medical College of Philadelphia in 1856. Male practitioners in Milwaukee published a false obituary of her in hopes that she would leave town, a threatening and resentment-filled gesture. In

1868 they rejected her for membership in the Medical Society of Milwaukee County, insisting that "the Society cannot survive the presence of a Woman."[13] Madison physicians did not form a medical society until 1886 and so could not exclude Anna from such an organization during her years in practice, but undoubtedly her male colleagues were no more happy to see her than were Wollcott's. Wollcott and Ott presumably knew of one another. They were the only female doctors in the state during the 1850s, 1860s, and 1870s, but no record indicates that they ever met.

This was not an easy time to be a female physician, and each woman could have used support and friendship. Dr. Ott began her career at a time in which educational leaders, physicians, clergy, and the general public debated the prudence of higher education for women. Wisconsin citizens and legislators argued about whether or not to admit women, and if so how, to the newly opened University of Wisconsin. In 1863 the university began to admit women but in 1867 shunted them aside to a separate Female College with its own curriculum. In 1875 university leaders again changed policy to create a fully coeducational setting. When Lavinia Goodell sought admittance to the Wisconsin bar that same year so that she could practice law, Chief Justice Edward Ryan of the Wisconsin State Supreme Court resoundingly denied her application. "The law of nature destines and qualifies the female sex for the bearing and nurture of the children of our race and for the custody of the homes of the world and their maintenance in love and honor," he declared. Women who entered professions such as law (and, presumably, medicine) "are departures from the order of nature; and when voluntary, treason against it."[14]

Women's medical education remained particularly contentious, despite long histories of white, enslaved, and indigenous female healers. Indeed, in Wisconsin indigenous women served as skilled healers. Women who sought to be physicians in the mid-nineteenth century not only faced plain old sexism but also ran up against the argument that women's brains and bodies lacked the capacity to be a physician. If these women were not white, they encountered the racist devaluation of their capacity: excluded from much of education, considered deviant even as medical subjects, and subjected to neglect at best and physical torture via medical experimentation at worst. The medical profession, in a blend of patriarchal ableism, diagnosed women's bodies and brains as pathologically unable, unfit to practice medicine. Just as the Medical Society of Milwaukee County had rejected Dr. Wollcott, much of the medical profession nationally responded with immense hostility to women's presence.

In 1873, the very year of Anna's eventual committal and incompetency determination, the famed Harvard medical professor Edward H. Clarke published the now infamous but then very widely read *Sex in Education*. So popular that it went through seventeen editions in thirteen years, "two hundred copies reportedly sold in one day" at the nearby University of Michigan.[15] Clarke warned that women who engaged in sustained vigorous mental activity such as education risked sterility, masculinization, insanity, and even death. His work exemplified an influential wing of the profession armed with medical certainty that education and professional lives rendered women "violently insane."[16] Clarke built on Dr. Isaac Ray's *Mental Hygiene* (1863) and Dr. T. W. Fisher's *Plain Talk about Insanity* (1872). Fisher, quoted verbatim by Clarke, detailed the many educated women he had treated whose minds had been ruined by their education. He warned, "A certain number of girls are predisposed to mental or nervous derangement. The same girls are apt to be quick, brilliant, ambitious, and persistent at study, *and need not stimulation, but repression*" (italics added). The women most interested in education and the professions were those most susceptible to insanity and thus most in need of repression. Such repression, he insisted, was vital, because insanity due to female education would not manifest itself while the young woman attended school; instead, it would appear "after the excitement of school life has passed away."[17] Cloaking sexism as benevolent and healthful caretaking, Clarke and Fisher, like the Medical Society of Milwaukee County, excluded women. Feminists, female scientists, and women desiring a medical education argued forcefully against such ableist patriarchy.

Despite such skepticism and regardless of one's thoughts on female physicians, Madison residents needed medical care. Though in 1880 city promoters claimed "the almost perfect salubrity" of the area, treating malaria remained a standard part of Wisconsin medical care until the 1870s, just as it had been in Ohio.[18] Cholera, typhoid fever, dysentery, malaria, smallpox, burns, broken bones, and complicated births required the same care in Wisconsin as they did in Ohio. Potential patients would have either called at her home or sent a message asking her to attend them in their homes, just as they had done for her first husband, Dr. Jonathan Miesse. A medical need could arise at any time of the day or night. Across the state, few patients paid with cash: in 1880 a routine birth could be paid for with a small pig, minor surgery was valued at several hams, and an office visit could be charged at fifty cents or "three haircuts, half a duck, eight dozen eggs, a bushel of potatoes, or seven pounds of cheese."[19] Anna's nearly twenty-year unofficial apprenticeship with Jonathan, aided by the medical supplies he accused her of stealing in their final divorce record, prepared her to practice as well as or even better than medical school would have done.

Details on Anna's medical practice are frustratingly scarce. She delivered babies and had done so as early as 1857, indicating that her practice started nearly immediately upon her arrival in Madison in the fall of 1856.[20] The most substantive evidence of the details of Anna's practice is a $15.03 receipt for medical purchases made in 1872 from Dunning and Sumner, local "druggists and grocers." At that time, she purchased a surgeon's needle, some ether (an anesthetic), and adhesive plasters, indicating a practice that included surgical procedures. She also bought medicines, including bryonia (used to treat pleurisy and peritonitis), glycerin (from which she could have produced her own creams or pills), a "female syrup" probably used for menstrual pain, and savin (a form of juniper used for eliminating worms or parasites from the body and for inducing abortions).[21]

Whatever the size of her medical practice, Anna did well financially. Her earnings as a healthcare provider added to her financial and land investments. Her ongoing property purchases, including the building and land that housed George's tannery, provided rental income. The large acreages she had purchased throughout the Midwest did the same. Like many people in her time period, she also lent out cash at standard interest rates. This earned additional funds.

Financial success, of course, was not enough and did not guarantee a happy household. In January 1859, about two and a half years after their May 1856 wedding, nearly three years after Jonathan Miesse divorced her, Anna filed divorce papers against her second husband, George V. Ott.[22]

In the month before Anna filed for divorce the Ott household affairs had become so horrific that she had sought the assistance of neighbors. Per her later court filings, late one evening during a windy and cold Wisconsin winter snowstorm, George "forcibly expelled" Anna and twelve-year-old Aurelia from their beautiful new home and locked the doors against their reentry. (Minetta was not mentioned, which only adds to her mystery. Nor was approximately five-year-old George F. S. Ott.)[23] The word "expelled" matters, for if Anna had left of her own initiative, she would have been entitled to no economic support from her husband. If he "expelled" her, the courts could impel him to provide economic maintenance.[24]

The two sought refuge at the home of a neighbor family, where they stayed "for about ten or twelve days." One wonders how the family responded when Anna and her daughter banged at the door during a late-night snowstorm and if they had known of or suspected the violence in their neighbors' home.[25] Generally in this period "the first acceptable refuge of many battered women was with a father who could extend male protection," but Anna had no family nearby. She turned to the next commonly used resource: neighbors.[26] Sager has shown that "Wisconsin community members regularly engaged in these types of interventions" for neighboring women facing household violence in the late 1840s and 1850s.[27] This was the first of many examples of widespread knowledge of Anna's life as a target of her husband's violence.

Assured by George's promises that "he would ill-treat her no more" and again according to her later court filings, Anna and assumedly Aurelia returned to their home after nearly a week and a half. On the day after Christmas, however, George "again commenced to assault" his wife "and did then and there beat, kick, and otherwise violently abuse and ill-treat" her. That evening Anna sent for a local alderman "to procure his interference for her protection." Perhaps she sent a household servant, or perhaps Aurelia ran through the streets on the evening of the day after Christmas. The alderman's intervention may have helped in the short term, but the next day George again beat Anna while she was at his leather goods store (property rented from her). On December 29 he "forcibly and violently assaulted, and beat, bruised, and kicked, and otherwise abused her person." On the 30th he "seized this plaintiff by the throat and so held and choked her until she became insensible." Recovering "sufficiently strong to leave the house" by the next day, Anna once again took refuge with the same neighboring family.[28] The divorce complaint provides no evidence of what happened to Aurelia or of what the neighbors thought.

On January 5, 1859, Anna swore out her first divorce complaint. She asked that George pay her legal fees and "suitable maintenance" during the legal proceedings and that he "pay and restore the amount of money and valuables" he had taken from her and "converted to his own use." The complaint stated that since July 1857 (just over a year after their wedding) Anna had "seldom if ever at any time been free from the marks resulting from the continued ill treatment and personal violence" perpetrated by George. The document detailed fractured foot bones, a two-week confinement to bed due to a particularly horrific beating, and one event in which her head was beaten so badly that she "became insensible . . . was speechless and unable to recognize any person present and wholly insensible for several hours thereafter."[29]

The options before the court were limited, just as they had been for the local alderman whose assistance Anna had sought. Beating his wife and knocking her unconscious lay within George's legal rights as a husband. Local men might ostracize him, voice or express their disapproval via intimidation, or ignore or even encourage such violence. Circuit court officials must have given some credence to Anna's claims, for the judge ordered George to pay Anna's legal costs so that she could "carry on this action."[30] Given the involvement of both alderman and neighbors, presumably many members of Madison society knew of the Ott household's violence. People in Madison talked, just as had people in Chillicothe.

For reasons unstated, in February 1859 Anna dropped the divorce case and moved back into the home on East Wilson Street with George. Again. Presumably Aurelia did also. No evidence of George's voice, other than the forceful echoes of his persuasiveness, remains.

A hint of an explanation about the goings-on in the Ott household on East Wilson Street is in the 1860 census. When the census taker canvassed the neighborhoods of Chillicothe, Ohio, several states away, the household of Jonathan and his second wife, Elizabeth, included Aurelia. The young teenager Aurelia had returned to Chillicothe to live with her father, Jonathan Miesse. Perhaps Jonathan heard of Anna's attempted divorce proceedings or of the cold December night when his daughter was locked outside the house and called for his daughter's return. Or perhaps Anna feared for her daughter's safety and sent the child back to Ohio. Whatever happened, Aurelia left the Ott household.

The 1860s left only blurry archival hints regarding Anna Ott's life. In early 1861 the Civil War began. Many men left Madison in order to fight in the war, though George did not. The wartime service departures included several of Madison's physicians, and this undoubtedly left Anna's medical skills in higher demand. A prominent Madison attorney, William W. Tredway, who would later hold an important position in Anna's life, came to prominence as the solicitor general of Wisconsin, responsible for all the financial affairs and goods pertaining to military training, service, and veterans in Wisconsin. Neither Jonathan nor Cornelius served in either the Union or Confederate military.

In this period Anna suffered several losses. She likely missed Aurelia's presence greatly, though she may have been thankful for her daughter's safety in Chillicothe—a safety brought about not by her distance from the war but by her distance from George. In July 1862 Cornelius died while in New York studying medicine. In 1863 Anna's mother died. Whether or not Anna attended either funeral is unclear. Both took place in Ohio. If she did, she likely saw her ex-husband, Jonathan, and her daughter, Aurelia (and Jonathan's second wife). The family buried Cornelius in a cemetery on the bluff above Chillicothe, not far from where Jonathan would later be buried. A young sculptor who lived in Chillicothe, Dayton Morgan, created an ornate and large tombstone for Cornelius. In April 1866, after the war's end, Morgan married Aurelia in Chillicothe. It is unlikely that Anna attended the wedding.

Residents of Madison who stayed behind did not experience the brutal realities of Civil War battles, but they did experience significant loss. Many

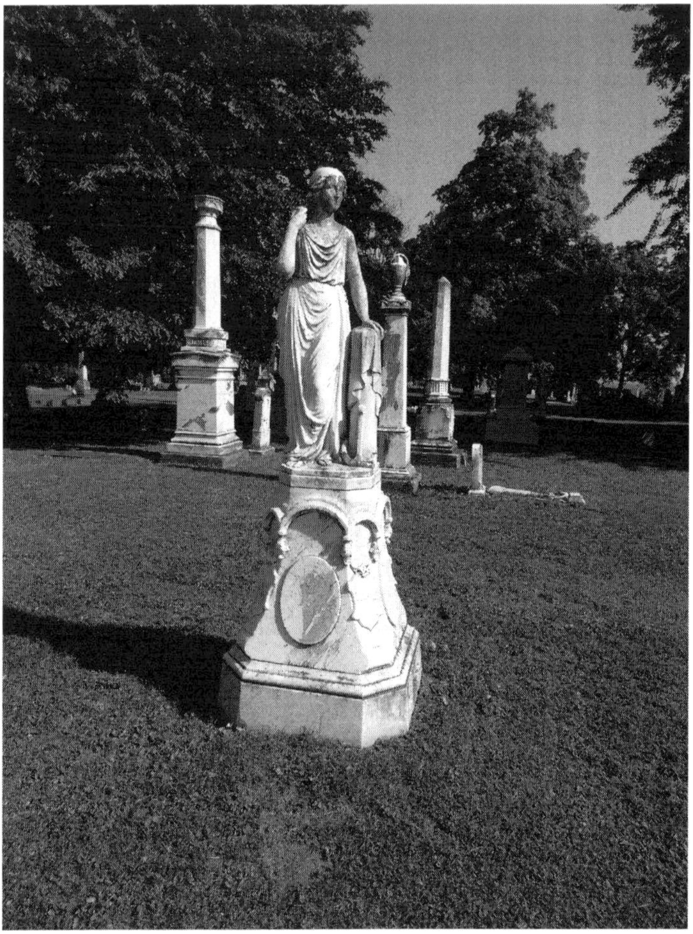

Image 2. Cornelius Miesse's tombstone. Photo by Kim Nielsen.

local men died. Many returned with bodies and minds mangled. Others, like Lucius Fairchild, returned with bodies altered, but they restructured successful lives with comparative ease. Fairchild, who lost an arm in the war, became Wisconsin's governor in 1866 and one of Anna's neighbors. Civil War chaos induced George, like many Union residents, to adopt creative economic measures. Due to wartime coin and gold shortages, he crafted tokens to give to customers who needed change when they purchased items. After customers accumulated a number of tokens they could return to the store to exchange the tokens for paper money or for goods. Even today, nearly a century and a half later, some of George's tokens remain among collectors.

After the war, Aurelia and her husband, Dayton Morgan, began to establish a life together. Early in 1868 the *Cincinnati Gazette* published a laudatory story on the "most modest and meritorious" sculptor Dayton Morgan. While Morgan resided at the Cincinnati Art School, Aurelia returned to Madison. Morgan's bust of Wisconsin governor Lucius Fairchild received artistic praise (which indicates that Morgan had visited Wisconsin), as did a bust of Aurelia. The *Cincinnati Gazette* described the artistic rendering of Aurelia as "a work of love in the double sense of the word—a love of art and a love of the subject."[31] In March but while back in Chillicothe, Aurelia gave birth to a daughter, whom she and Dayton named Hattie. Anna became a grandmother at the age of forty-nine. It is likely that Jonathan, and not Anna, delivered the child. Anna likely missed both her daughter's marriage and her granddaughter's birth.

In 1868 things once again began to fall apart for Anna. In June of that year, while still a new grandmother, Anna and her actions became entertainment fodder for newspapers across the country. On June 10, 1868, Anna chased a woman down a main Madison street while attempting to beat her with a horsewhip. Deborah A. Smith, a Civil War widow and dressmaker with two young sons, lived above Hawke's General Store at 78 Pinckney Street. Anna owned the building. George's store sat on the same street.[32]

Headline writers loved the story: "A Female Doctor Thrashes a Widow," "On the Rampage," and "The Doctress and the Horsewhip." Newspapers reported that "jealousy" motivated Anna but provide no indication of what that meant. A *Madison Journal* article reprinted throughout the country reported with relish that "Mrs. Dr. Anna B. Ott" had "visited Mrs. Smith's residence, told her she had come to have a settlement with her, and drew forth a horsewhip, and commenced applying it to Mrs. Smith's shoulders." Smith attempted to escape by running onto the sidewalk. Anna continued to strike her until several bystanders interfered. Anna then "put the weapon under her arm and went home," a walk of only a few blocks. The "considerable excitement" attracted significant attention. George was out of town, but if he had been at work in his store, he would have been close enough to hear the commotion.[33] It is hard not to wonder if George was enjoying the sexual company of the widow woman who lived near his store, but no evidence indicates this.

The next day Anna appeared before a local judge, pleaded guilty to assault and battery, and was fined twenty-five dollars plus court costs. When she "made further threats against Mrs. Smith" the judge cautioned her about possible additional fines. The newspaper articles that appeared across the country found Anna quite ridiculous, and presumably so did many of the residents of Madison. The *Cincinnati Enquirer* reported the news, so residents of Chillicothe also likely read and gossiped about the former wife of their local physician.

From the vantage point of a historian, it is easy to sensationalize but difficult to understand this event. The paucity of other historical sources of any kind, particularly those generated by Anna, amplifies the news story. What it meant to Anna, however, and how the community of Madison and George understood it are unclear. Similar male violence would certainly not have prompted the same level of attention, scorn, or ridicule. Courts and medical professionals later pathologized Anna's violence and used it as a weapon against her.

In late December 1868, nearly ten years after first filing for divorce from George, Anna initiated a divorce against her second husband for the second time. The remaining records are again frustratingly elusive but indicate tremendous turmoil between 1868 and 1873. Between December 14 and December 23, 1868, Anna lived in a local boardinghouse; she had been chased out of her home, she testified, by George's violence. She returned home, she insisted, only because she had no access to the money required to pay for her lodging and because George had promised that "if she would come back he would never strike her again and that he would settle her property honorably and satisfactorily." As the divorce proceedings progressed, whether or not Anna and George had "a cohabitation" (sexual intercourse) in the weeks after she returned on December 23 became a point of contention. Anna said no. George said yes. Anna later indicated that upon her return George had "commenced his tyrannical and abusive course toward her, as bad as ever. That he has since then treated her most cruelly, and that she has now the marks of his brutality upon her."[34]

The divorce case became one about violence and money. Once again Anna alleged that George beat her, and George alleged that it was all in self-defense against Anna's unreasonable and unpredictable behaviors. Anna alleged that George stole her funds and, as his leather business resided in a building owned by her, refused to pay the rent he rightfully owed. George alleged Anna to be selfish and greedy but denied none of her monetary allegations. Wisconsin divorce law, like that of Ohio, required a guilty party. If Anna's attorney could prove that she had gone to the boardinghouse or neighbors because George had "expelled her from the house" rather than leaving of her own accord, he would be obligated to provide alimony.[35] The case moved slowly between 1868 and 1870.

Anna's complaint alleged that several times a year, throughout their entire marriage, George had "upon the slightest provocation, and often without any, attacked her with his fists and knock[ed] her down choked her and kicked her shut her up threw her out of bed refuse[d] to provide for her support as a man as his circumstances should do and abused her in the most gross and insulting manner." The complaint claimed that George "is getting worse and more violent in his attacks upon her," and Anna now "fears for her life and cannot longer with safety live with him as his wife."[36] Anna's repeated efforts to seek refuge in the homes of neighbors and her repeated sojourns in local boardinghouses make clear that she felt unsafe in her own home throughout the couple's years in Madison. The household events must have been common knowledge among the town's approximately nine thousand residents, for she often left home to escape her husband.[37]

Violence and its various expressions in Anna Ott's life, whether as wife or institutionalized manic or in her mere shadow of an archival existence, should haunt us as scholars and human beings. The rhetorical description of household violence detailed in her divorce complaints reflected legal strategy, but all evidence indicates that such violence was Anna Ott's life. As Marisa Fuentes has said about sources pertaining to the very different context of slavery in Barbados, "To sit with these sources requires the capacity to hold and inhabit deep wells of pain and horror."[38] The combination of legalese and descriptions of repetitive, tedious violence makes Ott's legal complaints both hard to read and legally blasé. For example:

> And the plaintiff further shows that during the last spring in his own house he pushed her back into a corner of the room and near a bureau and upon and over the bureau and nearly broke her back and while in that position he struck her over the head with a rocking chair with such violence as to break it and cut around her badly from the effects of which she was sick and sore for a long time—and suffered great pain. That on several occasions since that time he has struck and beaten the plaintiff with his fists, and on the 1st day of December he attacked and beat her most brutally with his fists and made her eye discolored and made severe and painful bruises upon her head, and hurt and abused her so that she could scarcely stand, that he knocked her down insensible upon the floor and had to administer water to restore her to sensibility—from the effects of which beating she is still suffering and is so weak and injured that she can scarcely move and attempting to do so has fainted.[39]

As historians looking back nearly a century and a half later and as people who live in a culture with continuing and overwhelming domestic violence, we must hold and reread these life stories, even while their pain and horror are filtered through legal language. The marriage between George and Anna, like all such relationships, involved two people. Patriarchy, legal traditions, courts, community tolerances for violence, the privileges of money and status, sexism, and the weight of stigmatized diagnoses, however, went far beyond George and Anna. Her class privileges provided short-term escapes to a boardinghouse and may have influenced community perception somewhat, but they did not shield her from George's violence. Anna's later medical diagnoses and legal cases interwove this violence into their edicts, reflecting the complex relationship between ableism and patriarchy. The household and structural violence that pummeled her pummeled many.

Anna's attorney devoted the bulk of the 1868–70 divorce complaint to financial details and allegations. While court officials undoubtedly considered the violence horrendous or at least distasteful, once again the legal reality was that unless George were to kill Anna, there was little the court could or would do. As legal scholar Reva Siegel has noted, during the Reconstruction era courts "routinely condoned violence in marriage."[40] The court had legal grounds to respond and would have been more likely to act if George had robbed Anna of her money or goods. It thus made sense for Anna's attorney to focus on finances.

This complaint specified the existence of an antenuptial agreement. Anna and her attorneys insisted that before entering into the marital contract, she and George had signed an antenuptial agreement in which George had "agreed that she should have and control her own property after her marriage the same as before and that he was not to have any right therein." George and his attorneys never contested this point. Anna went on to say that after moving to Wisconsin, George had "by various ways induced" her to "let him have the use and control of it." She insisted that she had "never intended thereby to part with the titles and control."[41]

The divorce complaint began by establishing that Anna owned "in her own right . . . property of the value of at least ten thousand dollars and a very extensive and valuable quantity of gold and silver ware for table services." With those funds she had purchased property on Pinckney Street and taken "a deed therefore in her own name," and the balance "she used and kept separate from her husband." Anna had invested greatly in their magnificent home and its substantial lot, expecting that she "owned a joint interest in the house," but George had "obtained the deed in his own name without her knowledge or consent." Since 1862 George had run his business out of the lot and building she owned on Pinckney Street but had refused to pay her rent. When asked to do so, he would "abuse her in a most brutal manner."[42]

Anna and her attorney insisted that George had "managed to get the possession of" property valued at about $25,000 to which Anna was "legally and equitably entitled." George, they alleged, had left his wife with no income "with which to support herself." By violence and deprivation he "trys [*sic*] to prevent her from asserting her rights in getting her possession and control of her own property." As a doctor, Anna earned "large sums of money in the practice of her profession," but George had taken all these earnings and added them to his own wealth.[43]

George and his attorney had a different story. As he had in Anna's divorce complaint a decade earlier, George insisted that "each and all the allegations in regards to his cruel and inhumane treatment of the plaintiff . . . are all purely imaginary and entirely false." As he had in Anna's divorce complaint a decade earlier, George insisted that everything was Anna's fault. Though he had "not at all times been able to get along peaceably and happily" with her, what force he used was "necessary to prevent injury to himself or the wanton destruction of property," and any injuries resulting to Anna were "solely due to her own violence and desperation." Her behavior "was notorious to all the people of Madison."[44]

George then introduced interwoven allegations of Anna's insanity and unwomanliness, tying ableism and patriarchy together, echoing antisuffrage language that emphasized suffragists' physical unwomanliness, and pathologizing Anna's bodymindedness. George's deposition stated that Anna was "an unwomanly, large, muscular, masculine woman of violent and uncontrollable temper, and subject to strange and unaccountable freaks, at times almost amounting to insanity." He noted that after using the whip on Mrs. Smith, Anna had "kicked and struggled in the most unwomanly manner till she was overpowered." He complained that, "contrary . . . to the propriety of her sex," she had "frequently come to the store and spent much time there, espousing authority, and interfering with him and his business." When he had taken "occasion in a friendly way to tell her that she ought not to be there interfering in the store" Anna "flew into a rage." She "seized a pole and went to smashing the glass partition between the front and back front of the store." She struck at George with "both hands full of some bridle bits . . . but he pushed them back and held her fists for a while" and "held her for some time and tried to reason with her and induce her to become herself." After George let her go, "she jumped up and about, accusing him of murdering his first wife, burning his tannery, and everything else she could think of, and then threw a dish of dirty water over him."[45]

George offered this event as "a fine specimen of the plaintiff's conduct in her rages." During such occasions she was simply and in all ways unwomanly. Despite George's best efforts, he could not induce her "to become herself."[46] The nature of George's bodymindedness, unremarked upon by either him, Anna, or any attorney, is telling and signified power. Her body and mind were inseparable, boiled down to a deviant and insane unwomanliness. His unremarkableness as a white man who behaved appropriately as a husband was the norm against which she was measured and pathologized.

Accusations of unwomanliness, particularly for a woman of Anna's class, had legal power. Historian Leslie Harris argues that "if a woman failed to behave properly" in cases of marital violence, "she became 'unsexed' and violence was justifiable." In 1856 a Wisconsin court had ruled that one woman's conduct decades earlier had been "most wanton, most wicked, and most disgraceful"; thus, her husband's violence was legally defensible. This woman had cut her hair short, dressed in men's clothing, and taken a boat from Milwaukee to Cleveland. Her "desexing functioned as *de facto* justification for abuse, even though the abuse occurred years after this woman's act of rebellion." Though Anna was perhaps somewhat unsexed as a female physician, her class and educational status meant that others expected her to behave within relatively inflexible and specific womanly parameters. Serving as a physician might be tolerable. Responding physically to the assaults of her husband, even if they were true, was not.[47]

George sought to place himself in the best light, as Anna did. He insisted that he had "continually endeavored to make the best of his lot," treating Anna "with kindness and affection." There was, he and his lawyer claimed, "no settled antipathy between the parties" but instead "much mutual liking that would ordinarily be thought compatible with the occasional occurrence of scenes like those above described." If Anna would only "live and act like other women she might live as happily as others."[48] Like Jonathan had, George blamed his marital problems on Anna's gender deviance, her failure to "live and act" according to nineteenth-century norms of white femininity.

Having dismissed the violence as Anna's fault, George, like Anna, went on to discuss finances.

But stop. Hidden in George's deposition are tantalizing details. In the lengthy details George provided about what must have been a horrendous scene at the tannery is his mention of Anna's accusation that he murdered his first wife, Anna's youngest sister, Sophia. The complaint filed by George's attorney stated that Anna "jumped up and about, accusing him of murdering his first wife, burning his tannery, and everything else she could think of, and then threw a dish of dirty water over him." George and his lawyer did not have to include the details of this accusation, and by including it, they apparently thought it of no consequence. As a reminder, the historical record that remains provides no evidence of the date, location, or cause of Sophia's death. Whatever was true or not true about the narrative of violence George relayed in his deposition, his perplexing inclusion of this seemingly inconsequential detail indicates that Anna likely had accused him of murdering her sister. If she believed it, she believed that she was living with, was married to, and had reason to fear her sister's murderer. If she believed it, she believed that her nephew, George F. S. Ott, by then a teenager, lived with a father who had murdered his mother.

George did not contest the existence of Anna's separate property but claimed that she had "always . . . manifested a constant greediness" about property. She kept her "doctoring" money to herself, even though he had provided a horse and buggy for her use. He paid her taxes and expenses, but despite that, she had "frequently taken money from the store" and added it to "her separate property." George maintained that Anna had "a considerable sum hid away" in banks outside of town. Furthermore, he claimed that "within the past two or three years he has met several large losses" and thus could afford neither the divorce nor the cost of an attorney. It was, George and his attorney maintained, "a matter of justice and equity" that he not be required to pay for court costs, attorney fees, or anything in a divorce settlement.[49]

Striking is George's understanding of marriage, incorporated by his attorney into the divorce petition. George insisted that within their marriage, despite all, lay "mutual liking" and that such "mutual liking" was "compatible with the occasional occurrence of scenes" like the violence and anger described in great detail and length as occurring in the public arena of the tannery. Perhaps George expected such tumult within all marriages, though this may have been his lawyer's rhetorical strategy to convince a judge that the violence and public scenes of the Ott marriage were normative. George insisted that upon Anna's return from the boardinghouse the two of them had "lived and cohabited and slept and eaten together . . . on the most friendly terms."[50]

But no evidence indicates a friendly household.

Finally, in this fourth divorce complaint including Anna, a third party testified for the first time, and testified to George's failings as a husband. Margaret Stein, a domestic servant who worked in the Ott household, insisted that she had "never seen anything to make her suspect" that the two had been "together as man and wife." When George was in the house, Stein testified, he was "cruel and ugly to her [Anna] and has not shown her any kind of affection. Almost all the time when in the home he has been scolding her and abusing her and Mrs. Ott has frequently cried." Stein noted that George locked Anna out of her bedroom (they slept in separate rooms), denying her access to clothing and goods, "even a change of clean under clothes," and locked up "provisions," denying her access to food. George locked her blankets and bedclothes in the storeroom. In addition to denying bedclothes and blankets during a Wisconsin December, George "refused to allow a fire to be built in [the] furnace since that he has kept the house cold and uncomfortable and refused to have [a] fire built for the purpose of warming the part of the house occupied by Mrs. Ott."[51] Stein affirmed Anna's truth.

The judge, who likely either knew or had heard of both husband and wife, sided with Anna. In late January 1869 he ordered that George pay all legal fees and provide a monthly living allowance. George also had to vacate the store building owned by his wife. He had to allow her access to their home to take clothing and "medicine used by her profession" (again, a recognition of Anna's medical status in the community). George must, the judge insisted, "postpone" selling his wife's personal property and "refrain from interfering with her personal liberty."[52] In other words, George could not profit by selling Anna's material goods, and he could not lock her up. George must have vacated the storefront owned by Anna, for throughout April 1870 she advertised the building as available for rental.[53] In December 1870, two years after filing for divorce, she once again dropped her divorce suit.

Reading through the legal documentation that emerged from the Anna and George Ott household from 1856 to 1870, it is easy to forget that children lived in the household during these years, for they are never mentioned. Both George F. S. Ott and Minetta Monona remained connected to the household. Aurelia left around 1860 but occasionally visited, and she lived there once again with her two-year-old daughter, Hattie, in 1870, but had gone by 1874. The courts never asked these children or young adults about the violence in their household. Assumedly, all were very aware of and likely even the victims of the violence in their home.

George and Anna's life from the time she withdrew the divorce suit in late 1870 until the summer of 1873 remained relatively legally dull. At some point in these years, Anna's granddaughter, Hattie, died.[54] In the summer of 1871, a domestic servant sued the Otts for defamation and lost wages. In the summer of 1872, Anna's father, Ulrich, died. Anna inherited additional funds, but how she learned of his death and the extent of her contact with her family are unclear. None of the historical records remaining from the time Anna moved to Wisconsin until after her death indicate any communication with family beyond her daughter, Aurelia. Anna's isolation from family continued to grow.

The brief lawsuit of 1871, however, merits more attention. Former Ott household domestic servant Josephine Waldschaky, only seventeen years old, jointly sued both Anna and George (in that order), claiming that they owed her unpaid wages. She also charged that Anna had defamed Waldschaky's character by telling others that she was "a common strumpet, a loose thing" who had robbed Anna to "obtain the means to procure an abortion" and was "in the habit of going to bad houses."[55] She asked for compensation of $5,000. Anna testified that Waldschaky had stolen property valued at $476. The attorney representing the Otts defended them by saying that Anna was insane. Anna's "defamatory words," the attorney argued, had little or no impact because they were spoken while "under any mental derangement." The jury found for Waldschaky, finding that the Otts owed her $450 in unpaid wages and $68.36 in court costs but ignoring her claims that Anna had defamed her. The strategic use of insanity as a legal defense apparently provided the Otts some financial protection but rendered Anna vulnerable. This legal defense is the first mention, at least in the archival remains, of insanity.

Approximately a year later, in the spring of 1872, the Wisconsin governor, Madison city promoters, and members of the local elite hosted the national gathering of the Association of Medical Superintendents of American Institutions for the Insane (AMSAII). For local physicians, the gathering of prestigious physicians from across the country offered a unique opportunity.[56] Over forty insane asylum superintendents and assistant physicians met in Madison for their annual meeting from May 28 to 30. AMSAII attendees invited local "members of the medical profession" to join them each day, introduced several who did so, and spent one afternoon "visiting the excellent arrangements of the State Hospital for the Insane." Upon completion of their meeting they passed a resolution praising the "wisdom and discretion" of the hospital's leadership. The reputation of the city, the state, and the state's relatively new Hospital for the Insane benefited from the positive publicity this event generated in medical journals and newspapers locally and across the country.[57]

The AMSAII proceedings make clear that the professionals in attendance were male. The "ladies accompanying them" went on boat and carriage rides, attended receptions, and at least once "honored" the gentlemen with "their presence" while the men deliberated important topics.[58] Local physicians may have been welcomed, but Dr. Anna Ott was not.

While attending physicians spent significant time debating the causes of insanity (physical defect? heredity? trauma? a combination?) and whether or not insanity pleas had a legitimate role in the courts, they also shared concerns and strategies regarding two issues they believed threatened their power and their profession nationally. First, nearly all institutions reported overcrowding. For example, the superintendent of the Jacksonville, Illinois, asylum reported routinely having one hundred more patients than he had room for, resulting in people sleeping on the floors and in the corridors. A California superintendent reported having two to three hundred people regularly sleeping on the floors. Another physician testified that the institutions in which he had served had never *not* been overcrowded and pointed to a Massachusetts hospital built for 250 that held 470 residents. The Mendota asylum was similarly overcrowded, even though it had opened as recently as 1860. All hoped that the spring 1873 opening of an additional state asylum (in Oshkosh) would alleviate the problems, though that opening was a year away. The physicians attending the AMSAII could not agree on the causes of insanity, but they unanimously passed a resolution stating that insane asylum overcrowding was "an evil of the greatest magnitude" and against "the best interests of the insane."[59]

The other issue concerning AMSAII members was more complicated and less easily addressed than the thorny issue of overcrowding: state legislative proposals to protect the insane, sometimes called personal liberty laws or Packard Laws. In the 1860s and 1870s, in the words of historian James Mohr, a "national crusade against unjustified incarceration further discredited the flagging asylum movement."[60] Former inmates published numerous exposés of maltreatment and abuse by asylum personnel and family members who sought to institutionalize them for economic or personal gain. Propelled by sensational exposés and stories of economic malfeasance, state legislatures across the nation began investigations into insane asylums. Iowa and Illinois passed legislation guaranteeing jury trials and/or due process prior to commitment, as well as mail privacy while institutionalized, and they sought to insure that asylum inmates knew their rights. Other states, as well as Congress, debated such measures.[61]

Elizabeth Packard stood out nationally as the most prominent and effective advocate for the rights of those institutionalized as insane and as the author of the most widely read exposé. Packard had disagreed publicly with her Calvinist minister husband by siding theologically with Methodists. As her biographer, Linda Carlisle, wrote, "What Packard viewed as resistance to oppression and standing up for her rights her husband viewed as 'perversity of behavior' and evidence of insanity."[62] Illinois law allowed husbands to commit their wives to insane asylums with virtually no due process other than the word of the husband. At the initiative of her husband, Packard remained confined in an Illinois insane asylum from 1860 to 1863. As she wrote, "When once in the Asylum I was beyond the reach of all human aid, except what could come through my husband, since the law allows no one to take them out, except the one who put them in; or by his consent; and my husband determined never to take me out, until I recanted my new opinions."[63] Packard left the asylum committed to campaigning for legislation protecting the inalienable rights of those considered insane. Then, discovering herself unable to regain access to her children or property, she also sought legislation protecting the rights of married women.

Though men participated in asylum reform efforts, women led these campaigns and generally understood them as simultaneous campaigns against patriarchal abuses. While they did not use the word "ableism," these women understood how ableism and patriarchy intersected. In 1861 suffragists Susan B. Anthony and Elizabeth Cady Stanton explicitly linked asylum abuses to laws disadvantaging women and claimed that many women were locked away because they rebelled against male power: "Could the dark secrets of those insane asylums be brought to light . . . we would be shocked to know the countless number of rebellious wives, sisters and daughters that are thus annually sacrificed to false customs and conventionalisms, and barbarous laws made by men for women."[64] Elizabeth Packard linked lax commitment laws and the legal limitations of married women as she campaigned for "personal liberty laws" across the nation. The ease with which husbands could commit their wives, she argued, created examples of "legal kidnapping." In her case, it was "a wicked plot against my personal liberty and my rights."[65] She entitled her 1870 best seller *Marital Power Exemplified in Mrs. Packard's Trial and Self-Defense from the Charge of Insanity; or, Three Years Imprisonment for Religious Belief, by the Arbitrary Will of a Husband, with an Appeal to the Government to So Change the Laws as to Afford Legal Protection to Married Women.*

While those attending the AMSAII meeting knew of such activism, Dr. Mark Ranney, who at the time was the superintendent of the Hospital for the Insane in Mount Pleasant, Iowa, and then later became the superintendent of the Wisconsin State Hospital for the Insane, brought the issue directly to the attention of the 1872 meeting.[66] Some in attendance had lost jobs or faced scrutiny because of such activism. Those in attendance understood the Iowa Act to Protect the Insane as a direct threat to their authority, and they were correct. The Iowa legislature created a separate board with the power to inquire into why individuals were committed and confined to the insane asylum and how they were treated, and the board could fine or even imprison asylum employees who detained residents illegitimately.[67] Ranney and those present blamed the success of such legislation on the "indefatigable" efforts of Elizabeth Packard and her "grossest misrepresentations" of life in an asylum.[68]

The Iowa board consisted of a physician, an attorney, and "a lady." The "lady" particularly concerned AMSAII members. They questioned if she was "reliable" and if she engaged in "communication" with Elizabeth Packard. Someone asked, "Is she a woman's rights woman?" Upon this question the esteemed physicians dissolved into laughter. The gentlemen then adjourned. They joined "the ladies" for an "afternoon excursion" on Lake Monona and spent the evening at "the hospitable residence" of the Wisconsin governor.[69]

Anna undoubtedly knew of this event. She was well aware of the laws both enabling and restricting married women. She also knew that her husband's attorney had called her insane only a year previous in order to win a lawsuit filed by a former domestic worker. This was not a professional world welcoming to a woman such as her.

Then Anna attempted to vote. Anna obviously knew of Wisconsin suffrage activities, limited as they were in this period. In February 1869 Susan B. Anthony, Elizabeth Cady Stanton, and Mary Livermore had spoken to a "densely crowded" audience at the state capitol, urging the legislature to adopt universal suffrage. In 1870 Wisconsin suffragists met in Janesville for a convention led by Stanton.[70] Whether or not Anna attended either of these events is unknown, but she clearly followed national suffrage debates. During the presidential election of 1872, suffragists across the nation, including Susan B. Anthony, claimed their right to vote by simply attempting to do so. The resulting legal case surrounding Anthony remains a pivotal step in the expansion of the US electorate and an important example of civil disobedience.[71] On Election Day in 1872 Anna attempted to vote at the Third Ward's polling location, using the widely deployed suffrage argument that as a tax-paying citizen she should be able to vote. Those administering the vote said no.[72]

After Anthony voted she reported with enthusiasm to Stanton, stating that "not a jeer not a word—not a look—disrespectful has met a single woman."[73] Anna left no record of her experience, but another Madison-area woman voted with a much less positive experience than Anthony's. According to a letter written to the local newspaper by "A WOMAN CITIZEN," the election supervisor "looked daggers" at her as she entered "into the presence of the Board [of Supervisors] and heavy fumes of smoke." After pontificating on the rights of "male citizens," the board chair rejected her vote. She left, looking forward to the day when the town board had brains unaffected by "tobacco smoke" and "lager beer."[74]

Anna likely had a similar experience. Despite this, no evidence of her involvement remains in any Madison or Wisconsin women's organizations, and this omission is jarring. She appears isolated. Dr. Laura Ross Wolcott of Milwaukee, the other Wisconsin woman believed to be a medical school graduate, played a pivotal role in the state suffrage organization.[75] Female physicians across the country exercised leadership in many suffrage and reform organizations on local, state, and national levels. It would have been natural for Anna to do the same. She had funds and substantial property of her own long before the state legislature granted other Wisconsin women the right to control their own earnings in 1872.[76] Others believed her to be highly educated, and she practiced successfully as a professional when few other women did so. Perhaps she did not want such engagement or was embarrassed by the violence of her household. Perhaps other women rejected her presence because of her household. Perhaps they dismissed her as insane.

Regardless of what others thought, Anna attempted to vote in 1872. She sought this political agency despite hostility and despite her multiple vulnerabilities. As a local physician, as a woman of financial wherewithal, and simply because she wanted to do so, she sought to shape her own life and to have an impact by whatever means she could.

6. Anna Ott, Insane Asylum Inmate

IN MAY 1873, just six months after Anna had attempted to vote, George admitted her to the Wisconsin State Hospital for the Insane. The couple likely came by horse and buggy. The trip from their home would not have taken long, for the route along the shores of Lake Mendota to the large state institution was less than two and a half miles. May weather in Wisconsin is unpredictable. Perhaps the sun was shining on lilacs and trilliums; perhaps it was cold, wet, and windy. No indication remains of whether or not Anna knew of her imminent institutionalization. With the assistance and signatures of two of Anna's male physician colleagues, George had filled out and signed the paperwork the previous week. Anna became patient number 1763.[1] Medical experts determined her to be insane, and judicial officials determined her to be legally incompetent. The prescriptive results of her stigmatized medical diagnosis included and went beyond institutionalization to include the legal processes of guardianship and divorce. The forceful combination of legal and medical authority kept her at the Mendota Asylum until her death in 1893.

Identifying the messy array of historical forces whirling around Anna's institutionalization complicates the ableist pathologization of her life. According to George, she was unwomanly. In the larger community, her professional status and money privileged her but also marked her as unusual, a deviation from the norm. Her institutionalization occurred simultaneously with powerful national debates about women's biological capacity to become professionals, debates that wove patriarchy and ableism together, and amid local knowledge of her unusual behaviors. Her institutionalization also occurred during the growth of feminist activism. She sought authority over her own resources, safety, and public life while in a marital relationship widely recognized as violent, and she sometimes did so in unconventional ways. Like all women married to violent men in this period, Anna lacked structural supports; unlike many women married to violent men, she had no nearby familial resources to draw on, for the rest of her large extended family remained in Ohio. Medical and legal authorities characterized her body and behaviors, her very bodymind, as pathological and aberrant. In addition, violence lay not only at the core of her individual marriage but also at the heart of institutionalization, patriarchy, and the settler colonialism from which she profited. A complete analysis requires wrestling with this structural and historical mess and acknowledging the unevenness by which analytical frames map, and fail to map, on individual human lives.

The messy combination of historical forces that precluded Anna Ott's institutionalization followed her inside the hospital's walls of long-lasting brick and stone. The 105-acre site, also referred to as the Mendota Insane Asylum, was not an insulated place apart. From its very beginning the hospital became and remained woven into the community's economic, legal, and social structures. It reinforced the establishment of settler colonialism and literally walled in whites deemed incapable of relating with family or neighbors appropriately, managing self, managing goods, or productively laboring. The institutional walls became both literal and metaphorical building blocks for patriarchy and ableism, aided the regional development of capitalism, and were used by state officials as proof of the state's advancement. Individuals, money, material goods, and the fruits of labor moved back and forth between the asylum and the community, replicating and reinforcing larger social structures. Nineteenth-century asylums were horrible places in which to be confined, but within that context Anna exercised great privilege.

Legislators and hospital staff noted the 1860 opening of the Wisconsin State Hospital for the Insane with pride. Before even opening its doors, its leadership proclaimed optimistically that "the fact is now universally recognized, that insanity, if appropriately treated at an early day, is curable." Institutional personnel thus encouraged state residents to refer insane individuals as soon as possible, for the hospital could hold only three hundred people.[2] The hospital's first residents entered in July 1860, and by the end of the year seventy-eight remained. Eleven had been discharged as cured, and three had died. The first superintendent declared the institution "already a success, which the people of Wisconsin may contemplate with pride and pleasure."[3]

The hospital's architecture and staffing reflected the most up-to-date medical expertise of Dr. Thomas Kirkbride, one of the founders of the Association of Medical Superintendents of American Institutions for the Insane (AMSAII), superintendent of the Pennsylvania Hospital for the Insane, and a leader in the "moral cure" movement (also known as "moral treatment").[4] Kirkbride and other national leaders of the AMSAII believed that humane treatment, a therapeutic regime of work and leisure, and the coercive measures of drugs and institutional confinement could cure insanity. Kirkbride espoused limited if any use of physical restraints. Physical restraints, however, remained a contentious issue in the field, and some superintendents strongly advocated their use. Mendota superintendents used physical restraints at higher rates than the national average. Between 1840 and 1880 the number of psychiatric institutions in the United States expanded from 18 to 139. The majority of new institutions, including Mendota, used an architectural plan created by Kirkbride.[5] As the size of institutions grew, superintendents struggled to match their therapeutic ideals with institutional realities.

Daily practices in the Wisconsin State Hospital for the Insane reflected this national trend. Governing the ever-growing institution and its people, maintaining the building and grounds, and enacting the moral cure provided the superintendent and his staff with a considerable challenge. The main building was four stories high; it contained kitchens, storerooms, reception rooms for staff, visiting rooms for inmates, offices, staff accommodations, dining rooms for staff that varied according to rank, and a large chapel. The three-story wings were sex segregated. The first story housed domestics and attendants; the second and third stories had wards for inmates. Each floor had six single lodging rooms, a dormitory for four patients, a parlor, a bathroom, a water closet, a lavatory, a clothes room, a drying room, a soiled clothes hopper, and a dust flue. The institution was no small endeavor.[6]

Just five years prior to Anna's 1873 institutionalization and only eight years into the institution's life, the 1868 suicide of a patient from a well-respected family, complaints about economic malfeasance, and rumors of brutal treatment prompted the Wisconsin legislature to investigate conditions at Mendota. The resulting 716-page report harshly criticized Superintendent Abraham Van Norstrand for encouraging the abuse of patients and profiting by selling to the state hospital defective supplies at inflated prices from a business owned by himself. These sales left asylum inmates with rotten eggs and moldy halibut.[7]

The 1868 Wisconsin congressional committee detailed three major problematic findings regarding the treatment of those institutionalized as insane in its widely publicized report. First, they found that both asylum attendants and the superintendent placed inmates in isolation as "a common practice," using "a strong dark room usually without furniture of any kind save, perhaps in some instances a bed or a straw mattress on the floor." This room was variably referred to by staff as a "strong room," a "blinded room," a "dark room,"

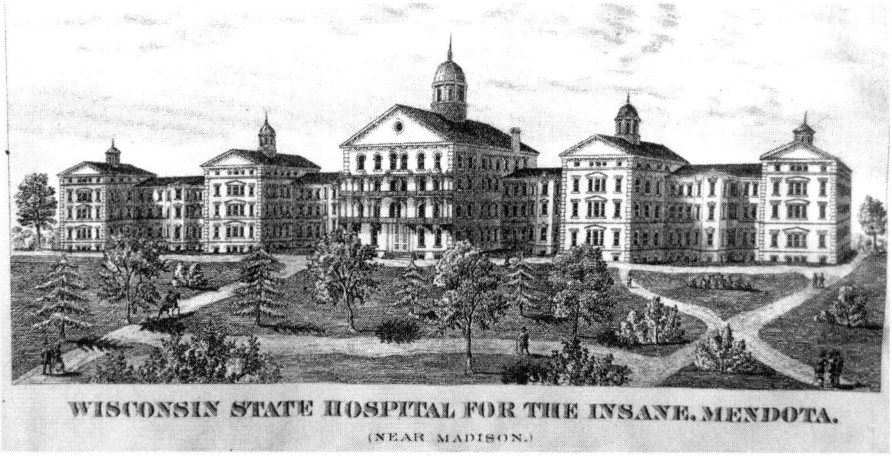

Image 3. Wisconsin State Hospital for the Insane, Mendota. Wisconsin State Institutions, Lithographs, M99-119, Wisconsin Historical Society.

or "a shuttered room." Second, they found that Mendota staff used physical restraints at higher rates than did staff of other asylums across the country. Finally, they concluded that "cuffing, slapping, kicking, striking, pounding and choking are common if not daily practices in the treatment of the patients by the attendants." The congressional committee called for Van Norstrand's dismissal (he resigned before they could fire him) and concluded that at the Wisconsin State Hospital "kind words, loving acts, gentleness and a tender regard for the comfort and well being of the patients" had been replaced by "harsh words, cruel deeds, roughness, brutality and a total disregard of the comfort and well being of the unfortunates here confined."[8]

In an appeal to the public, the 1868 legislative committee asked Wisconsin citizens to imagine their own "mother, sister, wife or daughter" as a "helpless woman, bereft of reason." She might, they feared, "be strapped to a seat with her hands in a muff or confined by a strait jacket, utterly incapable of inflicting any injury upon any one." Along might come the superintendent, "a large powerful man," and the beloved family member "in her helpless, irresponsible condition spits on his clothes." In the scene, the superintendent "raises his heavy hand, and in his angry passion inflicts blows on the side of her face and head that leaves the face black and blue!"[9] In this public imagining, the physician was male, the vulnerable patient was female, white, and helpless.

Anna Ott was someone's mother, sister, wife, and daughter, and as a community member and a local physician, she probably had heard and read about the 1868 investigation and its findings. Perhaps she had even attended one of the hearings, for the capitol was only a short walk from her home. Perhaps she had even visited a patient at the asylum.

The intake questionnaire completed by George in 1873 indicated that Anna's insanity was hereditary in nature (proven by the existence of an insane maternal aunt). The "malady" had first manifested itself just two years prior and was increasing. Anna was well educated, both prior to her immigration to the United States and as a "graduate of a physician and a medical college in Philadelphia." George claimed that Anna had delusions that included the fear that "all men are conspiring to obtain her property." He said she frequently threatened both suicide and homicide.[10] The prior (and later) divorce records raise questions about several of George's answers. His claim that he had "only tried to quiet and soothe her with words" should, at the very least, be questioned. And while the restraint and confinement referred to in these questions likely referred to the use of a medical device called the crib (to be explained later), the court's direct order to George to "refrain from interfering with her personal liberty" during the 1868–70 divorce attempt indicates that being locked up was not a new experience for Anna.[11]

Around the same time as Anna's institutionalization, two other white women of relatively high status, Elizabeth Packard (1860–63) and Mary Todd Lincoln (1873), were also institutionalized after widely publicized diagnoses. Male family members initiated both women's institutionalization. Packard decried the nearly unlimited power of husbands and physicians to institutionalize wives. She linked lax commitment laws and the legal limitations of married women as she campaigned for personal liberty laws across the nation. The ease with which husbands could commit their wives, she argued, created examples of "legal kidnapping," in her case, "a wicked plot against my personal liberty and my rights."[12] Similarly, Lincoln's attorney publicized unjust institutionalizations and critiqued the expansive power of asylum superintendents.[13] As explained earlier, feminist activists understood the cause of asylum inmates and the cause of women to overlap and to be entwined. Both Illinois and Iowa passed laws in the 1860s establishing rights of appeal for those institutionalized.

As activist Elizabeth Packard had alleged, white families found it relatively easy to commit family members and particularly easy to commit female family members. Illinois law only required that a person be "evidently insane or distracted" and had relaxed procedures for the commitment of married women in 1851.[14] At the Pennsylvania Hospital for the Insane, widely recognized as the leading institution in the United States, Superintendent Kirkbride originally required one physician's testimony. When state legal changes required the statement of two physicians in 1869, Kirkbride considered it a threat to the judgment of physicians. As historian Nancy Tomes said of the Pennsylvania Hospital for the Insane, "As long as the doctor and the family agreed upon the verdict of insanity, the difficulties in judging borderline cases rarely led to public controversy. The only party likely to challenge the doctor-family consensus, that is, the patient, had little power to dispute the decision."[15] At the Utica, New York, State Lunatic Asylum family members initiated 75 percent of commitments in this period.[16] Wisconsin law required a certificate of insanity from two physicians.[17]

Whether or not Anna knew of these cases is unclear, but the superintendents of asylums certainly did. Dr. Mark Ranney, who became superintendent of the Wisconsin State Hospital for the Insane in the summer of 1873, worked with other superintendents to oppose such activism. At the 1872 AMSAII meeting in Madison, Ranney had blamed the success of such legislation on the "indefatigable" efforts of Packard and her "grossest misrepresentations" of life in an asylum.[18] Packard's activism challenged the authority of asylum superintendents and husbands. It is likely that George also knew of these legal and legislative debates.[19]

During the rest of that summer, Anna's medical records included only four additional entries. Such a level of documentation was not unusual. On June 24, 1873, staff noted that between June 12 and 24 she had been allowed to visit "town" twice. Though no indication was made of where she went or what she did, the attending physician indicated that she had become "quite refractory because we would not allow her to visit her home."[20] Perhaps she had desired clothing, books, or medical supplies, or perhaps she wanted to check on her garden. Perhaps she simply wanted to remind herself that she had a life outside the asylum. Her "trip" to town was not unchaperoned and self-determined.

Outside the grounds of the hospital, while asylum personnel characterized Anna's concerns about her property as "fiercely fixed delusions," George petitioned the court to declare Anna legally incompetent and thus to give control of her property and finances to a court-assigned guardian. If declared legally incompetent, Anna could not sign legal documents, make decisions about spending or investing her money, sue or be sued, or make any legal decisions. She would have the same legal and fiscal standing as a minor. At this moment, her economic resources did not help; indeed, they rendered her more vulnerable.

Once again, Anna's voice is found only by reading between the lines. On July 19 Anna's husband, George; her nephew and stepson, George F. S. Ott (by then age twenty); and the local judge visited her in the hospital. They focused on the task of identifying a guardian, not on whether or not one was needed, and assumed that the court would find her to be incompetent. While Anna technically had no say in the assignment of a guardian, she must have had opinions on this issue, for, as the medical records indicated, the group "could come to no understanding as to a guardian."[21] In this period in Wisconsin, courts overwhelmingly appointed husbands (occasionally wives), sons, and other male relatives as guardians. Non–family members became guardians only as a last resort. The standard court procedure would thus have been to appoint either her husband or her stepson as Anna's guardian. Anna clearly did not want either one as her guardian and the legal controller of her property. She may have threatened to contest the guardianship if such was the court's ruling, for she had fiscal means to hire a lawyer and do so. Perhaps George wanted to be appointed guardian. The judge's willingness to engage Anna in this discussion suggests a willingness to take her seriously—perhaps due to sympathy for her, perhaps in consideration of the violence she had previously encountered, or perhaps because of her financial wherewithal.[22] The judge's willingness to engage her in this discussion, despite her diagnosis of insanity and the pending determination of incompetency, also suggests that while he went along with her diagnosis and confinement, he still believed her to have capacity. Patriarchal ableism had its practical side, which is not the same as kindness, and it was not all-powerful.

Though still lacking an agreement about a guardian, on July 24 the local court formally accepted George's petition to have Anna declared incompetent, and the Dane County Circuit Court judge set a court hearing date of August 14. The court ruled that Anna be served a copy of the order and, "if able to attend be produced at said time and place of hearing."[23] She had a legal right to attend the hearing.

A week prior to the hearing Anna's physician complained about her in institutional medical records. She was, he wrote, "very fault finding and difficult to please, and interfering with treatment of patients." Interfering with the treatment of patients! Dr. Anna B. Ott must have felt herself capable of judging other physicians at the State Hospital for the Insane and expressed that judgment. She was both patient and doctor. The hospital physician also noted more about Anna's delusions. At this time, when she knew of the possibility that she might lose all control of her property in the forthcoming hearing, the physician noted that she "imagines all the City authorities are in league against her to obtain her property and to defraud her generally and also that the laws of the land and of God are false and specious."[24] Anna had clearly been voicing her opinions about her upcoming incompetency hearing.

The day before the hearing, Judge George E. Bryant received two letters lobbying for Anna's incompetence. Superintendent Ranney wrote to the judge insisting that she not be present at her hearing, a disregard of the law and simultaneous resistance to growing national legal trends that limited the authority of asylum physicians. Six local physicians and all the "respectable citizens of the city," the doctor claimed, could testify to Anna's insanity. Forcing Anna to listen to such testimony, he insisted, would produce "an alienation of feeling" that would render her more "unpleasant." Dr. A. J. Wandsum, a local Madison physician, also submitted his determination of Anna's insanity. "She is insane," he wrote to the judge, specifically with "monomania."[25]

Judge Bryant ignored this lobbying. Anna's medical records indicate that on August 14 she was "taken over to town today to take part in having a guardian appointed."[26] Judge Bryant insisted that Anna had the right to be present, and perhaps she likewise insisted on it. She attended the hearing. What Anna said, or if she said anything, is lost, for documentation regarding what went on at the hearing no longer exists. Despite or because of her presence, the Dane County Probate Court determined Dr. Anna B. Ott legally incompetent. On September 5, 1873, the Dane County Probate Court named W. W. Tredway as the legal guardian of Anna B. Ott.[27] The three-week span between the incompetency hearing and the appointment of her guardian suggests that determining a willing guardian agreeable to everyone took work and that Judge Bryant engaged in such work. As judge, he could have appointed anyone. Tredway was a wise choice, and his appointment as guardian significantly shaped Anna's next decades.

William W. Tredway (1804–89) had settled in Madison in 1858 and quickly risen to legal and social prominence. During the Civil War he had served as Wisconsin quartermaster general, in charge of purchasing and dispersing all necessary military goods, ranging from clothing, food, and tents to guns and ammunition. In this position he had responsibility for over a million dollars. After the war he was made responsible for ensuring that Wisconsin's Civil War veterans received the pensions to which they were entitled. Tredway had a reputation for honesty, good financial management, and civic responsibility. In a town the size of Madison in 1873, if George and Anna did not know him, they certainly knew of him—and vice versa. All available evidence indicates that Tredway managed Anna's monies honestly and in ways that allowed her power and (limited) autonomy.[28]

When Dr. Alexander McDill, then superintendent of the Mendota Insane Asylum, admitted Anna to the institution in 1873, he diagnosed her to have "a diseased brain," specifically, "chronic mania with frequent exacerbations."[29] The state hospital's statistical register noted Anna's diagnosis simply as "mania."[30] Experts considered mania a form of "uncontrollable or furious madness where behavior was violent, frenzied, boisterous, or delusional."[31] Thomas Kirkbride of the Pennsylvania Hospital for the Insane treated mania with both drugs and moral treatment. Morphine, he argued, calmed those with mania and weakened their delusions. Kirkbride supplemented morphine with "cups or blisters applied to the back of the patient's head or neck, warm baths with cold applications to the head, and mustard foot baths" to reduce the excitement believed inherent to mania.[32]

Asylum superintendents such as McDill developed diagnoses based on their reading of medical manuals, consultation with other physicians, and prior diagnostic experiences, and they were taught that they could discern insanity by looking at their patients. Prominent US physician Benjamin Rush, whose medical guidebooks were still widely read at the time of Anna's commitment, had written in 1818 that "women, in consequence of the greater predisposition imparted to their bodies by menstruation, pregnancy, and parturition, and to their minds, by living so much alone in their families, are more predisposed to madness than men."[33] Dr. T. W. Fisher's 1872 *Plain Talk about Insanity*, a widely used text, described mania as "an excessive and expansive activity of the mind" that included often violent and extreme action. According to Fisher, maniacs directed their energy outward, with "exhilaration, extravagance, exaltation, expansion, exaggeration, explosion."[34] In his widely used 1883 guidebook for physicians, Dr. Allan McLane Hamilton noted that brain diseases had "well-marked bodily symptoms." Hamilton warned that while all asylum inmates possessed "repulsiveness . . . this is especially the case in the female." Insanity, he insisted, caused women to "rapidly lose their good looks . . . and plainness or downright homeliness is the rule." The suspicious, violent nature of the manic became embodied by an "averted head and sinister expression," "a contracted brow," and "deep and sharply drawn lines around the mouth." The chronic manic female, who usually looked downward, would sharply draw up her head upon meeting others and begin swearing, cursing, and shaking her fist. She would wear "a scowl," "a contemptuous sneer or a malicious grin." Hamilton also warned of delusions of grandeur, obscenities, coarse hair, and "carnal allusions."[35] McDill would have looked for these physical and behavioral traits as he diagnosed Anna. At Mendota, physicians disproportionately diagnosed women with mania. For example, in 1877, 58 percent of those diagnosed with (uncategorized) mania were female; 63 percent of those diagnosed with any specific kind of mania were female.[36] Across the nation, 38 percent of those institutionalized as insane held the diagnosis of mania in 1880.[37]

Only one other individual entered the state hospital on the same day as Anna: a thirty-nine-year-old white man diagnosed with melancholia. One month prior, Wisconsin's newly opened Northern Hospital for the Insane (near Oshkosh) had begun accepting patients.[38] Most of them were transported by train or buggy or on horseback from the overcrowded state hospital on Lake Mendota. Anna thus entered the hospital at a time of relatively low inmate population. The other people institutionalized in May were diagnosed with insanity due to wide-ranging factors: "religious excitement" (two residents), "unknown," "did not get school," "hereditary," "dissipation," "epilepsy," "injury of head," "previous attack" of insanity, "intemperance" (alcohol usage, three residents), "jealousy," "masturbation," "death of parents," and "puerperal" (due to childbirth).[39]

Like all private and public asylums built in a wave across the nineteenth-century United States, the legitimacy and authority of the Wisconsin State Hospital for the Insane rested on acts of diagnosis. Diagnosis is a powerful act. It is a rhetorical magic wand. It casts specific bodies and minds as pathological and in need of cure—and it casts other bodies and minds as desirable. When diagnosis is sought or claimed, such as by those in the nineteenth century who identified themselves as melancholic or insane, it could be empowering and justified claims to resources. Embodying or having a diagnosis is thus a powerful way of being that ostensibly defines one's needs and indicates one's future. Diagnosable behaviors and diagnosable embodiments are thus of potentially significant impact and perform significant cultural labor. Furthermore, Anna Ott did not simply receive a vague diagnosis of little or temporary consequence. She received a deeply stigmatized diagnosis that furthered her civic illegitimacy. She lost all legal property rights and faced physical containment. Despite the prenuptial agreement she forged, despite the financial resources she had shrewdly acquired and the property she owned, despite her whiteness, her diagnosis marked her as unfit for civic, monetary, and marital participation.[40]

Across her lifetime Anna experienced diagnosis in multiple and complex ways. While she was the wife of a physician, diagnosis served as the economic and social center of her household. As a physician, her acts of diagnosis reaffirmed her social status, generated an income, and reflected the privileges of an education others believed her to hold. Being the recipient of a stigmatizing diagnosis, however, was very different. A mania diagnosis propelled her into a new space literally and figuratively. Her diagnosis generated physical boundaries that removed her from the community where she had practiced for over fifteen years and confined her to the asylum grounds. Unlike a diagnosis of influenza or a broken limb, the diagnosis of mania recast her social legitimacy. Anna's medical diagnosis of mania, a kind of insanity, and her legal diagnosis of incompetence, interwoven with the numerous other historical forces and individual circumstances of her life, denied her ability to know and tell the truth and rendered any claims she made illegitimate. The diagnosis reduced her to an easily dismissed and ultimately ridiculed madwoman and made impossible any moral high ground she may have hoped to be able to claim as a white wife and victim of male violence. Despite the financial resources she had shrewdly acquired, mania marked her as unfit for civic and economic life and ended her professional career as a physician. Yet, as will be shown, diagnosis was not all-powerful, and it leaves us with a messy analysis for which Anna exercised, and others allowed her to exercise, some economic control.

Stigmatized and pathologizing diagnoses did not and do not simply happen. The diagnosis (mania) and prescriptive treatment (institutionalization) that Anna received came from somewhere and someone. She did not *receive* a diagnosis as she would *receive* a present. Nor was she *given* a diagnosis in the same way that someone would *give* her a present. In these cases, language hides the active historical agents. Diagnoses' claim to science and thus ahistorical grounding rendered invisible the individuals who issued them, who acted behind the claims of expertise, and the historically situated nature of diagnoses. Anna's diagnosis and its corresponding prescriptive treatment were enacted by individual people and reinforced by powerful social structures. Her husband, George, state hospital personnel, local physicians, and the county probate court judge diagnosed and then institutionalized her, buttressed by the local medical community, the national context of the medical profession's growing power, the growing power of law and the region's court structures, and the reliance of white Wisconsin residents upon the emerging structures to insure their settler-colonial strength. Diagnoses and prescriptive treatments frequently reflect and reinforce a multitude of powerful, intersecting, sometimes apparent and sometimes less so social forces. That is the case whether the diagnosis is of healthfulness and vigor or of a pathologized state of being.[41]

Of those institutionalized in the same month as Anna, no one remained as long as she did. The melancholic male who entered with her left four months later, in September. The last was gone by 1889; ten had left due to either "recovery" or "improvement." Hospital staff discharged four as "unimproved." Five left the institution the same way Anna was to do in 1893—in a coffin.[42]

Putting together the pieces of Anna Ott's daily life within the walls and grounds of the Wisconsin State Hospital for the Insane on the shores of Lake Mendota is difficult. The grounds of the large institution were and are beautiful. Anna's money and the acquiescence of her guardian, Tredway, in letting her spend it largely as she desired made her institutionalized life easier than it otherwise would have been. Twenty years in the Wisconsin State Hospital for the Insane, however, meant twenty long years of institutionalization and confinement.

The hospital superintendent held responsibility for all that happened within. State legislatures and professional standards directed superintendents to supervise all medical care and maintain correspondence with the family members of inmates. They also had responsibility for all the buildings, industry, and grounds. At the four-hundred-acre Mendota site this included farm animals, clothing production, amusements, and things such as, in 1884, an unexpected die-off of over five hundred wheelbarrows of fish in Lake Mendota (even more damaging, in the area of the lake used for drinking and cooking).[43] The duties of the superintendent, in the words of Superintendent McGill, were "perplexing, onerous, and never ending."[44] While the nationally respected Dr. Thomas Kirkbride oversaw the private Pennsylvania Hospital for the Insane for forty-three years, superintendents of public institutions tended to have substantially shorter tenures. During Anna's twenty years of institutionalization, nine superintendents led the Wisconsin State Hospital for the Insane. At least two were driven out by investigations into economic malfeasance and administrative failures. Their stay varied from four to sixty-five months, with an average of twenty-two months.[45]

Assistant physicians thus often conducted what direct care occurred. Historian Ellen Dwyer found that in New York institutions, by 1860 superintendents had "allocated most direct patient care to assistant physicians."[46] These were demanding positions. As Dr. Isaac Ray wrote of the ideal assistant physician in 1873, "His heart is in his work, and no call to recreation or rest can draw him away from it. To him the hospital is father and mother, brother and sister, sweetheart and wife."[47] Mendota generally had two assistant physician positions, with significant turnover.

The staff members with whom inmates such as Anna had the most contact were the attendants, who had responsibility for the "immediate and constant care and supervision of the patients."[48] Hospital superintendents required attendants to "make beds, scrub floors, and bathe filthy patients, [while] they also expected them to offer moral guidance and psychological counseling."[49] Ideally, attendants would render "every attention needful for the bodily comfort, and by unceasing acts of kindness soothing the troubled spirit." While superintendents tended to praise attendants publicly, privately they complained about them, often blaming the predominance of Irish immigrants for the supposed laziness, irresponsibility, and low intelligence of attendants.[50] Attendants worked long hours for poor pay with little control over their lives, resulting in constant employee turnover. At the Utica asylum, "attendants worked fourteen to sixteen hours a day" in this period and had time off limited to "a half day once a month, two evenings a week, and every third Sunday." Even during leave time they had to request permission to leave hospital grounds.[51]

Attendants at the Wisconsin State Hospital for the Insane were to perform "all duties that may be assigned to them" with "cheerfulness," "receiv[ing] suggestions and corrections kindly." They were to use no tobacco or alcohol and "avoid everything contrary to order and decorum." Bad behavior included "sitting on tables, lounging on settees, or heavy walking, hurrying up or down stairs, slamming of doors, loud talking, rude forms of address, profane and improper language, all vulgar habits, and every kind of act unbecoming [to] their position."[52] Attendants lived in the main building and were locked out if they had not returned by 9:00 p.m. In 1873 female attendants earned $167 per year, male attendants $260 per year. (In comparison, the hospital engineer earned $900 in 1873, the butcher $384.) Superintendent Ranney publicly complained of the low wages, telling the legislature that if it raised salaries, the institution could attract and retain a higher quality of attendant.[53]

In Madison, as around the country, attendants generally had bad reputations. The 1868 investigation into the state hospital found attendants guilty of routine violence: "Cuffing, slapping, kicking, striking, pounding and choking are common if not daily practices in the treatment of the patients by the attendants." Turnover was such that over seventy people filled a total of fifteen positions in just four years. The investigation also found, however, that one attendant was often left in charge of thirty to forty people. Superintendents, rather than seeing a patient every day as assigned, could neglect patients for as long as six or seven weeks. Attendants were characterized as drunkards, "persons who were profane, persons who possessed anything but good moral characters, and who possessed scarcely a single qualification for the place to which they were assigned."[54] Ranney accused attendants at the state hospital of skimming cream off milk meant for inmates in order to make butter, running around at night, and holding "disorderly and noisy gatherings" in their quarters. Reportedly, they even had a masquerade party in which some dressed up as the superintendent and his wife.[55]

The notations in Anna's medical record were likely made by either the superintendent or the assistant physicians. A month after she arrived, on

June 12, 1873, medical staff noted that since her admission "Mrs. Ott has been quite orderly and conducted herself with all propriety." She required no medication, slept well at night, and took pleasant walks in the daytime. Mendota staff interpreted this good behavior, however, as her attempt to "act shrewdly" to conceal "her real mental condition." Proper and orderly behavior only proved Anna's devious nature, for she remained "possessed of many fiercely fixed delusions."[56] Similarly, in March 1874 the superintendent made an extended entry into her medical record noting her recalcitrant and unpleasant behavior. She had, he noted, "conducted herself well" during her first months in the asylum, but her good behavior meant that she had simply "concealed her delusions to a great extent." Such misleading behaviors had been designed "to deceive those in charge of her into belief in her sanity." Her true insanity could not be hidden, however, and she had become "refractory, fault-finding, difficult to please, officious and violent."[57]

Anna's behaviors annoyed asylum personnel, and staff considered deviations from general agreeableness to be proof of her insanity. For example, the record for March 6, 1874, concluded that she was "fault finding, exacting, imperious, tyrannical, treacherous and untruthful. The result of course of a disordered mind."[58] On November 11, 1876, her physician noted that she was "more agreeable of late. But continues capacious [*sic*] and faultfinding." She quarreled, called other women "bad names," broke her chair, twice attacked specific attendants, and once had a "wild fight today with patients and attendants but soon quieted down again." When good, she was "ladylike."[59]

Particularly notable in Anna's case file are words of assessment and characterization: officious, imperious, ladylike, exacting, interfering, quiet, impudent, profane, and troublesome. However we interpret the case file, it is unquestionable that conflict existed between Anna and Mendota's staff members and quite possibly between Anna and other inmates. When her behaviors pleased them, staff called her "pleasant" and "ladylike." Coupled with "pleasant" were notations of her walks in the grove (which is still a beautiful place) and her attendance at institutionally sponsored amusements—"dances, chapel, picture shows etc." When Anna displeased staff she was "impudent," "abusive," "delusional," "willey [wily, *sic*]," and "troublesome." Behaviors leading to these characterizations are frustratingly unclear. The few details included in the case file were complaining about the food and refusing to wear a new skirt and then ripping it apart.

Hospital staff believed that Anna considered herself better than they, and this attitude infuriated them. They characterized her as "imperious and exacting," "disposed to officiousness," "cross and impudent," and "bitter and sarcastic."[60] Several times staff complained of her bossiness to them and other patients, for example, "Seems quite officious on the hall and inclined to direct some."[61] Dr. Anna B. Ott may have been in the institutional role of a patient, but she claimed authority and esteem according to what she believed she deserved. She had lived with great violence in her Madison household for almost twenty years, and she undoubtedly experienced sexism as a daily part of her professional life, but she also had lived all of her prior adult life with status and privileges. As the wife of Jonathan Miesse, she moved through her community as a well-to-do doctor's wife. In Madison, she claimed the standing of a wealthy female physician. She had been declared incompetent and institutionalized at the Wisconsin State Hospital for the Insane, but she still had more money than likely all the staff and other inmates, and she was a physician who was believed to have more education than all the staff except for the superintendent and one or two of the doctors. A messy array of structural forces left Anna both privileged and vulnerable, claiming power and experiencing coercion.

Local and asylum physicians focused great concern and attention on Anna's delusions, and the diagnosis of her words as delusions had consequences. The admission records detailed her "prominent delusion" to be a belief in "a conspiracy afoot to defraud her of her property."[62] In 1881, when asylum physicians testified to Anna's insanity in the divorce suit filed by George, they also noted her delusion that others tried to "imprison her falsely, deprive her of her liberty."[63]

Medical staff documented what they considered to be Anna's additional "delusions," though they rarely documented the content of such delusions. Most medical record entries were brief: "October 29, 1880. Cross and impudent, delusions."[64] Out of sixteen references to delusions, only two detailed the content. Once Anna complained that others had broken into her trunk, stolen her clothing, and returned the clothing dirty.[65] Another time staff noted that Anna "attaches evil to everyone and imagines Mr. Ott is confined in the basement and that we are all combined to rob her of her just dues."[66] Hospital staff disregarded both of these claims as delusions and provided them as evidence of Anna's insanity.

Given Anna's tumultuous life and relationships, the violence within her life, her institutionalization, and the determination of her incompetency, it also is not surprising that she would "attach . . . evil to everyone" and believe all were out to "rob her of her just dues."[67] Such beliefs were not delusional, they were her life experience. George Ott, however, was not confined to the basement of the Wisconsin State Hospital for the Insane. At this point in Anna's institutionalization George did visit the hospital occasionally, but whether he spent time with her or simply spoke about her with Superintendent Ranney is unknown.[68] The Ott marriage had included instances when George confined Anna to certain parts of their home or locked her out of the house. Perhaps Anna believed George was confined in the basement of the asylum, or perhaps she was referring to an incident when George confined her in the basement of their home, and a hospital staff member misunderstood.

Consider the diagnostic reach of labeling Anna's words "delusions" and thus symptoms of insanity. Anna alleged that others tried to steal her money and imprison her. Such supposed delusions included a great deal of reality. Due to the legal determination of incompetency, Anna had lost legal control of her money, though the analytical complication, as will be shown, is that her legal guardian allowed her to do with her money what she desired. Due to the diagnosis of insanity, she was contained in an insane asylum. It is also not implausible that others stole Anna's clothing, for her clothing likely was of better quality than most staff or inmates could afford. Even in the asylum, she undoubtedly enjoyed furniture of higher quality than that in the homes of nearly all the asylum staff. Legislative investigations of the Wisconsin State Hospital for the Insane in 1868 and 1880 detailed the nearly routine theft of inmates' material goods.[69] Insane asylum inmates routinely had their material goods stolen throughout the nineteenth century. Indeed, nearly every newspaper exposé, state investigation, and individual memoir about asylum life published in this period included claims of thievery. Asylum personnel sometimes stole the property of inmates for their own usage or to sell for profit. Other inmates stole property so that they could enjoy it, warm themselves with it, barter it, or use it to bribe someone. The diagnostic pathologizing of Anna's words as delusions, however, meant that whatever she said could not be truthful, and in circular logic, her purportedly untruthful claims legitimized the diagnosis. Anna's diagnosis by asylum physicians rendered her illegitimate to asylum personnel and, as will be seen, to community members of multiple generations. Regardless of whether or not Anna experienced realities that aligned with others', the deployment of her diagnosis by physicians and the larger community had tremendous consequences.

Diagnosing Anna's claims as delusions also undermined any critiques or challenges to larger power structures imbedded within her words or behaviors. Historian Susan Burch argues that diagnoses of insanity imposed upon indigenous people institutionalized at the Canton, South Dakota, Asylum for Insane Indians effectively discredited challenges they attempted against the power of the asylum's superintendent, the Bureau of Indian Affairs, Western biomedicine, or the US government.[70] Similarly, the diagnosis of Anna as insane effectively discredited critiques of her husband's patriarchal power to seek her institutionalization and the institution's ability to keep safe those in its charge.

Evidence indicates high rates of violence in Mendota and similar institutions as part of daily life. At the Wisconsin State Hospital, much but not all of that violence took place in the infamous Sixth Ward. Similar to other institutions, the wards at Mendota were numbered one through six; the Sixth Ward housed "the most disturbed and untidy patients."[71] Anna's records indicate that her placement in the Sixth Ward was for control and punishment. Just a few months after her arrival, someone (presumably the superintendent or assisting physician) noted that her behavior "could only be controlled by placing her in the wing of 6th Ward."[72] In October 1873, her "very ladylike" behavior meant that she got to access the Second Ward.[73] In June 1874 attendants moved her to the Sixth Ward after she "became very furious, storming all day, threatening."[74] In 1882 her record indicated that she "remains on 6th Ward" and was "delusional and continuing abusive . . . obscure and profane."[75] Where Anna spent her last years is unclear; the last reference to her ward placement was in 1883 and indicated that she had "no change whatever. On 6th."[76]

The Sixth Ward tended to be infamous among inmates, staff members, and families, though for different reasons. When Dr. S. B. Buckmaster became superintendent in 1884 he noted that the Sixth Ward included "the most disturbed and untidy patients" of the female wards and was overcrowded. Each night five to eight women slept on the floor. The overcrowding, he said, was "disastrous in many ways. . . . noise . . . [people are] more inclined to quarrel, and injuries are sometimes inflicted on those about them."[77] Presumably, attendants preferred not to work in such wards. Both inmates and family members expressed their concerns about the Sixth Ward. After Thomas O'Kelly ran away from the hospital in July 1873, he wrote to the superintendent, asking, "Please sir, send that $40 worth of clothes and my clothes that you have in the bloody sixth ward."[78] When an inmate named Fayette wrote to a member of her family named Angelina York that she had been placed in the Sixth Ward, York wrote immediately to ask, "What has been the matter with Fayette."[79]

Rose Trautman's 1892 exposé of her time in the Wisconsin State Hospital for the Insane focused particularly on the Sixth Ward, "the worst ward in the building," in which she felt she was placed as punishment. After she had been arguing with attendants, "four of the attendants seized me and dragged me by my feet, down four flights of iron stairs, my head and body bumping from one step to another. I was taken to the last cell on the right hand side of the sixth ward wing." There she was given doses of henbane (used as a sedative) via hypodermic needle and left in an environment "calculated to destroy the health of the patients. Food of the poorest quality; pitchy rosin toilet soap that closes up the pores of the skin; musty, damp bedclothes; damp under garments." The ward was, she believed, a "malaria pit."[80] She chronicled violence on the part of other Sixth Ward women, the attendants, and assistant physicians.

Sometimes, but particularly throughout late 1875, hospital staff characterized Anna as violent. Her August 4 record noted that she "had a wild fight today with patients and attendants but soon quieted down again."[81] After Anna twice attacked asylum attendants in December 1875, once causing "considerable injury," Superintendent Mark Ranney made the decision to place her in the crib.[82]

Many doctors in the emerging field of psychiatry believed that the crib, first used in the 1840s by the State Lunatic Asylum at Utica, New York, was a calming treatment for disturbed or violent patients. Inmates considered insane could be placed in the crib, sometimes referred to as "the Utica crib," for hours or for weeks.[83] The wooden slats allowed individuals to receive food and to urinate or defecate without having to be removed. The crib was only one form of manual restraint used across the country as part of treatment. Restraints included the crib, isolation in a bare and locked room, bed straps, sleeves, mittens, and a canvas suit (the equivalent of a straitjacket). Famed superintendent Kirkbride argued for using restraints only as a last resort and then sparingly, but other asylum physicians considered them essential to treatment.[84]

How long Anna remained in the crib is unknown. Her December 7, 1875, medical record noted the decision to place her in the crib. The next notation is from December 30: "Quiet since the above."[85] At the 1874 meeting of the AMSAII, Dr. Ranney had argued for the crib's effectiveness, particularly with suicidal patients, saying that its use "affords a full equivalent for watching or other supervision, and it is less liable to abridge sleep than any other measures affording the needed security."[86] Clarissa Lathrop, a woman institutionalized at the Utica State Asylum from 1880 to 1882, called the crib "an instrument of torture."[87]

In 1868 a Wisconsin legislative committee had criticized Mendota Hospital staff for using the crib at higher rates than other hospitals did. Practices apparently did not change. An 1880 state investigation revealed that at most times one out of every ten or twelve inmates lay confined in a crib, an "unusually large" number. (At that time, 580 inmates lived in the facility, which had a capacity of 500; there were approximately 58 cribs.)[88] The investigation also revealed that hospital records generally did not even note crib usage. Anna likely spent far more time in a crib and was restricted by other forms of restraints than asylum staff noted in her medical record.[89] When Dr. S. B. Buckmaster became superintendent of the Mendota Hospital in 1884 he abolished all forms of mechanical restraints, removing "from the wards every crib, muff, belt, camisole, anklet, and other form of restraining apparatus."[90] When a new superintendent began in 1890 he returned to using "slight restraints."[91] Like the rest of the nation, Wisconsin physicians could not agree upon the use of restraints.

The many white women who published chronicles of their time inside insane asylums in the late nineteenth century made three primary arguments, all circling around experiences of violence. First, they directly tied their confinement to women's legal disadvantages outside the asylum. As Tirzah F. Shedd wrote in her support of Elizabeth Packard's activism, "It may be a land of freedom for the men, but I am sure it is not for the married women!"[92]

Second, they chronicled ongoing violence, perpetrated by attendants, sometimes physicians, and other inmates. As Phebe B. Davis wrote in 1855, "I saw a concentration of evils in a condensed form." Sophie Olsen wrote of her great fear of the attendants: "I had always some expedient by which I could easily disarm her very wildest maniacs, but I could never disarm or tame their far more ferocious keeper." Davis had warned all women facing institutionalization to cut their hair short, for long hair made it "more convenient for them to get a quick hold."[93] Wisconsin conditions specifically hit the news in 1892 with the publication of Rose Trautman and Barbara Trautman's *Wisconsin's Shame: Insane Asylums or the American Bastille! The Narrative of the Kidnapping of the Misses Trautman*. The two sisters, both schoolteachers in Sauk City, Wisconsin, spent two years in Wisconsin's insane asylums (1888–90, first Mendota and then the Northern State Hospital in Oshkosh). *Wisconsin's Shame* chronicled immense abuse by attendants, limited access to heat and food, and disregard by physicians. Trautman noted being dragged by her feet naked down the hall of the Mendota Asylum. She claimed that after challenging the superintendent's treatment of another female inmate, "he threw me down, and, taking me by the hair, pounded my head, face down, until I was spattered with blood." Rose Trautman hinted at sexual assault, saying that "the indecencies practiced upon the patients by . . . attendants . . . would be sure to bring Anthony Comstock's censure on me for sending obscene matter through the mail." She found physicians to be of no help and said she frequently "swallowed many a bitter pill when I saw attendants abusing patients."[94] The memoir painted a picture of routine violence in which asylum residents sought to help one another.

The third theme of women's asylum writings was the uselessness of their complaints, whatever their nature. Some feared and experienced retaliation

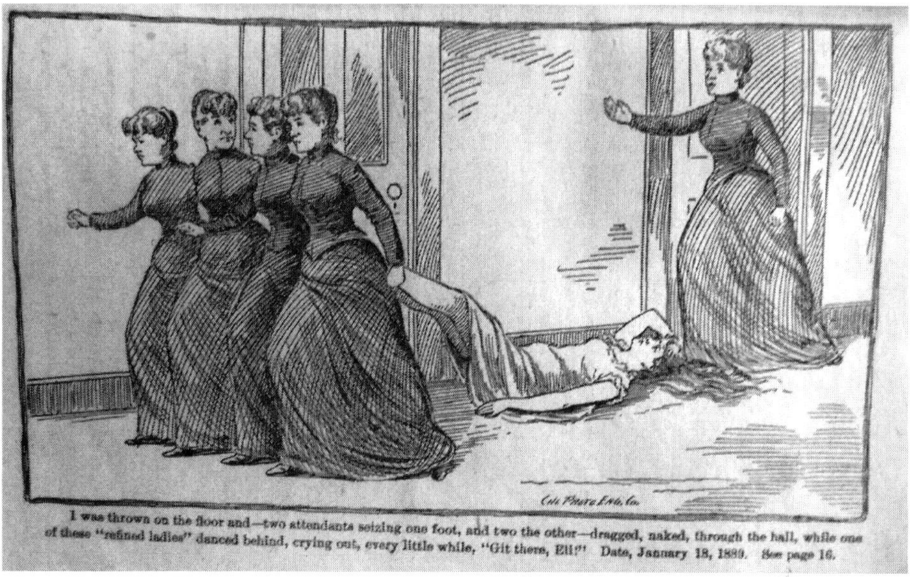

Image 4. A scantily clad woman is dragged by her feet by four female staff members. The text states: "I was thrown on the floor and—two attendants seizing one foot, and two the other—dragged naked, through the hall, while one of these 'refined ladies' danced behind, crying out, every little while, 'Git there, Eli!'" Rose Trautman and Barbara Trautman, *Wisconsin's Shame: Insane Asylums or the American Bastille! The Narrative of the Kidnapping of the Misses Trautman, of Sauk City, Wis., on a Sunday Afternoon, and Running Them into an Insane Asylum; Their Two Years' Shocking Experience and Observation in the State Hospitals at Mendota and Oshkosh* (1892), 17.

by attendants, saying it was "not safe for a patient to report one of the attendants."[95] Even more fundamentally, just as Anna's statements were dismissed as delusions, other institutionalized women found their words dismissed due to their diagnoses. Phebe Davis, who had been in the New York Lunatic Asylum, wrote, "When I said anything to the Doctors about the wrongs of the house, they would tell me that was my insanity. I told them that a fact was no less a fact because it was told by a crazy person."[96] The muckraking reporter Nellie Bly reported the same dismissal in her 1887 expose.[97] The famed reformer Dorothea Dix received similar responses from those in the emerging psych professions. In 1864 Isaac Ray, considered a founder of forensic psychiatry, warned Dix against believing as true the accounts of those considered insane.[98]

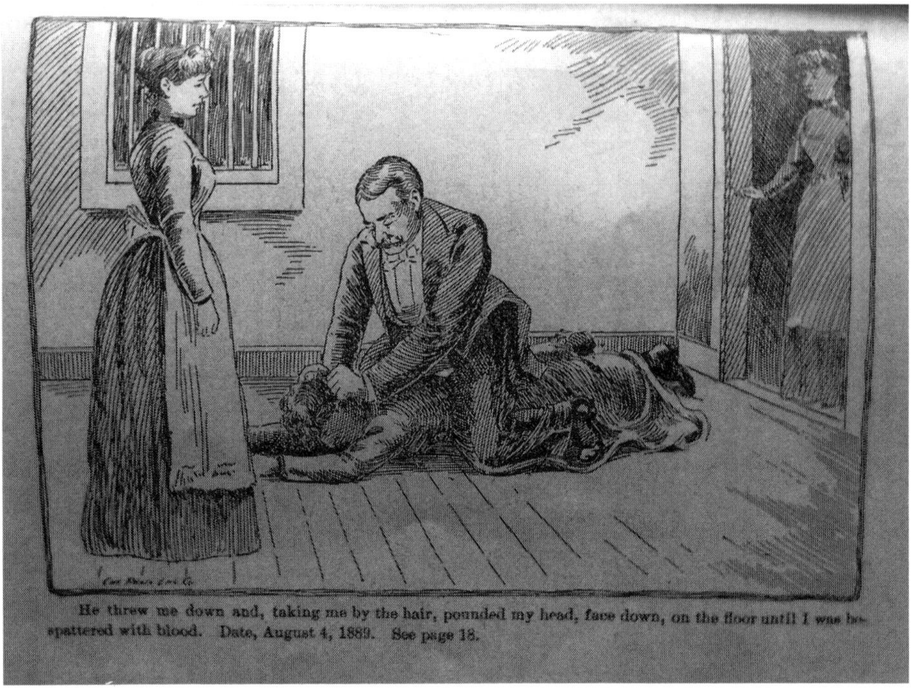

Image 5. A man sits astride a woman as she lies facedown on the floor. The text states: "He threw me down and, taking me by the hair, pounded my head, face down, on the floor, until I was bespattered with blood." Rose Trautman and Barbara Trautman, *Wisconsin's Shame: Insane Asylums or the American Bastille! The Narrative of the Kidnapping of the Misses Trautman, of Sauk City, Wis., on a Sunday Afternoon, and Running Them into an Insane Asylum; Their Two Years' Shocking Experience and Observation in the State Hospitals at Mendota and Oshkosh* (1892), 25.

The general strategy of members of the AMSAII was to dismiss such matters as illegitimate. They felt themselves under siege in this period and struggled with sensational exposés, letters, and memoirs written by former or current asylum inmates such as the Trautman sisters. State investigations, families seeking explanations of the suicides of their loved ones, and, most particularly, the activism and publications of former inmates claimed that such institutions were violent, chaotic, and poorly staffed and generally did far more harm than good.[99] According to AMSAII members, asylum residents were, by definition, insane. Therefore, what they said had to be unfounded or even ridiculous, a strategy similarly used by asylum personnel regarding

Anna's "delusions." Wisconsin State Hospital superintendents adopted this strategy in both 1875 and 1886: in 1875 the superintendent blamed criticism on "uncured patients and employees discharged for inefficiency or misconduct," and in 1886 the superintendent insisted that such "fabrications" hurt "prospective patients—patients who might well get treated early, and who would be committed early if friends did not so often hear these reports."[100]

Anna's purported acts of physical violence targeting patients and attendants took place within this larger debate and within larger violent structures. In August 1875, hospital staff noted in Anna's case file that she had "a wild fight today with patients and attendants but soon quieted down again." The December 1 and 7, 1875, records also noted that Anna attacked two female attendants.[101] Perhaps Anna initiated violence because she felt it was well-founded. Perhaps others initiated the violence and Anna received the blame. Sophie Olsen, who had spent a year in the Jacksonville, Illinois, Insane Asylum in the 1860s acknowledged that sometimes institutionalized women had "banded together in little secret societies, in earnest, agonizing consultation" about retaliating against confinement and specific staff members. She urged her readers, however, those who might "blame us for acting upon this," to "remember that we were fighting for our lives . . . that our lives were most essentially imperiled."[102] Anna may have felt herself similarly imperiled, similarly fighting for her own life and well-being. Her case file provides no substantial information about the violence noted within it. The violence of physical altercations had been a routine part of her life since she had married George Ott. She lived in a violent society of settler colonialism. State hospitals for the insane routinely included physical violence. Anna experienced violence under the guise of medical treatment when asylum staff placed her in the crib and, in 1885, when she spent two months receiving electric shocks (likely as a curative for paralysis, though they were also used to treat various forms of insanity).[103] Whatever the case, Anna's experience of medically prescribed institutionalization was that of being moved from one place of violence—her marital home—to another, moving from one kind of violence to another.

Much of the evidence used in this chapter, including that noting Anna's violent behavior while inside the asylum, is from her patient medical record (called a case file). Legal access to case files is complicated. In 1996 the US Congress passed the Health Insurance Portability and Accountability Act (HIPAA), a part of which seeks to guarantee the privacy of medical records. Largely intended to cover the present, HIPAA also has implications for historical scholars. Because I am a scholar, and because patient case files from the Wisconsin State Hospital for the Insane are held in the archives of the

Wisconsin Historical Society (WHS), I have limited access to these sources, and only with the permission of archival staff.[104] Given the amount of time since Anna Ott's death, and given my scholarly interest in a specific individual, I received access to her case file but hers alone. I neither sought nor received access to additional case files from this time period.

Ethical access to historical medical records also is complicated. Imbalanced power dynamics often characterized the relationship between an expert and a disabled person and thus shaped the primary sources resulting from such interactions. In addition, the coercive means by which many primary sources were created, collected, and maintained, especially some frequently used by disability and medical historians, is problematic. For example, many if not all of the photographs of Millie and Christine McKoy, conjoined twins born into slavery in 1851, made under the guise of medicine and science, were sexually exploitative, coerced, and sensationalistic. Photographs such as these, taken in a period and space in which African American women's bodies and disabled bodies were often coercively displayed and scrutinized, convey more about ideologies of scientific ableism/racism and those who perpetrated them than about the photographic subjects. Many people with disabilities live and have lived in times and spaces where they had no recognized right or access to privacy—privacy of body, privacy of space, privacy of information. Many people with disabilities lived in or moved in and out of spaces of coercion, incarceration, and institutionalization. Medical consent and bodily autonomy are modern notions; people with disabilities have been subjected to forced sterilization, medical experimentation, display, and sexual abuse. Case and medical records were laid open to those considered professionals but rarely to the individual involved. In all these examples, the less socially powerful an individual—men and women of color, white women, those of lower-class status, those considered sexually or gender deviant, targets of imperialism—the more vulnerable that individual was to the coercive generation of historical evidence.[105]

Using these sources, including medical case files, requires acknowledgment and careful consideration of our ethically fraught gains. I do not know if Anna Ott would grant me access to her case file. Would she even have imagined or dreamed that someone, a female scholar more than one hundred years after her death, would have sought that access? I am confident that she would never have done so. I am equally confident that the multiple asylum physicians who created Anna's case file would never have foreseen my historical consideration of their work.

Given these limitations, what might Anna's case file reveal? What does it actually reveal?

The first thing that is immediately obvious about the file is its brevity. This sparseness asserts less about the dismissiveness of asylum physicians and more about the extent of their responsibilities. It is easy to interpret the infrequent entries in Anna's case file (particularly when compared to the nearly hourly measurements of blood pressure in current hospitalization records) as physician neglect. However, the Wisconsin State Hospital for the Insane was originally built to house 250–300 patients, but in 1874 the daily average population of the hospital was 365; in 1884, 510; in 1893, 527.[106] Superintendents were supposed to attend to every patient every day, but with such numbers and with a superintendent's additional responsibilities, this was impossible even for the most dedicated and well-meaning superintendent. These ratios and responsibilities were the norm in late nineteenth-century public institutions, even as they resulted in neglect and disregard.

What we now would refer to as Anna's intake records are strikingly small when compared to today's medical documentation, and they largely repeated information that George had provided.

> No. 1763; Madison, Dane County. Admitted May 12, 1873. 54. Born in Switzerland. Married. One daughter 25 years. She is a physician. Attack began about two years ago. First attack. Cause of attack hereditary taint. Increasing. No natural intervals. She imagines that all men are conspiring to obtain her property. May injure others [during] some sudden passion. Has frequently threatened suicide and homicide. May tear clothing when in a passion. Cleanly. No treatment. Physical health very good. No confinement. Always very quick to anger. Temperate. No injury of head, etc. She has an aunt insane. Her parents were not related. Good education.[107]

Nowhere in any of these records is there a record of Anna's voice, though such an omission was standard practice. The narrators of her case file do not reveal themselves. The unquestioned authority of the case file cloaks authorship and the reality of ongoing personnel changes over its twenty-year span and presents its statements as omniscient declarations of truth. Most entries are two or three lines long. Sometimes there was a week between entries, sometimes as long as four or five months. From the perspective of over a century later, the case file, written to record and convey information about Anna Ott, reveals less about Anna and more about asylum personnel and life inside the asylum. From between the lines, however, evidence of her voice emerges—resistant and perhaps belligerent, definitely unhappy and angry.

Given the sparseness of the case file and given the time demands made upon physician superintendents of hospitals for the insane, the case file also reveals which details and conditions asylum personnel considered meaningful knowledge. "Facts"—such as medication, treatments, and the nature of the wound referred to on December 16, 1873—do not appear in the case file. Nor do details on what constituted "violent" and "abusive" behaviors. My historian self wants to know what, if anything, caused Anna to break a chair and a bowl (particularly when she herself had likely paid for them) in early June 1874. No evidence remains about what prompted a physician to write "fault finding, exacting, imperious, tyrannical, treacherous and untruthful" on March 6, 1874. Did the physician consider his authority questioned and therefore justify those characterizations by stating that such traits were "the result of course of a disordered mind"? The hospital physician considered it more important to note when staff moved Anna around the asylum from ward to ward. These moves were efforts to control her behaviors.

The major events in Anna's life went unrecorded in her file, which likely was the case for most if not all hospital residents. Aurelia's September 1879 visit to her mother went unnoted, though perhaps being reminded of her daughter was the reason for Anna's "bitterness" and "quarrelsomeness," chronicled vaguely around the time of the visit. Similarly, no record was made of Anna and George's divorce proceedings between June and October 1881. Indeed, no entries were made between June 1881 and January 1882. In the spring, however, she was noted to be "very bitter and sarcastic."[108]

After twice resisting Anna's efforts to divorce him, in 1881 George successfully sued her for divorce on the basis of her insanity. In 1881 the Wisconsin state legislature added insanity to the state's limited legitimate grounds for divorce, opening up new possibilities for George.[109] Divorce did not allow George to access Anna's financial resources, but it released him from all dower responsibilities (the setting aside of one-third of his estate for her support upon his death) and allowed him to sell land without having to provide bonds guaranteeing his wife's economic support. During the divorce proceedings, three local physicians testified to the incurability of Anna's insanity. One who had signed her committal papers in 1872 provided additional details about her life pre-institutionalization: "She was . . . very vivacious and talkative and with a great desire to manage her own business, and claimed to be and practiced and advertised as a female physician. She practiced a good deal. . . . She carried a pistol and said if she was interfered with she would shoot the first man that laid his hands on her." (This is the first and only mention of a pistol.) In this case, Anna's class, medical expertise, ambition, and pistol were used against her as part of the pathologization process. This physician used details of unconventional womanhood to add weight to his diagnosis of Anna's incurable insanity, establish her as a threat to men, and justify both institutionalization and divorce. Former Mendota superintendent Dr. Boughton testified to her insanity by detailing her delusions about imprisonment, the unchaste nature of "respectable people" in Madison, and the poisoning of food at the hospital.

When asked if George had contributed to Anna's insanity, a former state hospital physician testified with a logic that left Anna with no good options: "She complained that her husband had abused her but she never admitted that she was insane and so never claimed that her husband made her so."[110] In other words, one could not blame George for contributing to Anna's insanity because Anna would not admit she was insane. Thus she could not claim that he had made her so. Psychiatry at this time generally ignored the violence of husbands against their wives and its potential to have a traumatic impact.[111]

Multiple others testified regarding George's lack of responsibility for his wife's insanity and refuted prior allegations of household violence. A lawyer from the firm that had represented Anna in her two previous divorce attempts noted that "Mrs. Ott did not exhibit any marks of violence that I remember . . . she was either afflicted with lunacy or general cussedness to a greater or less degree." The Dane County sheriff, who was also the chief of police in Madison, characterized interactions between the couple as "hair pulling scrapes" and "a general family rumpus," testifying that he had never seen evidence of violence (apparently neither "hair pulling scrapes" nor a "rumpus" was considered violent); thus, "I therefore never believed her assertions of bad treatment but considered her an insane woman." George swore, "I never did her any violence except in restraining her and then did her no unnecessary violence as I believe."[112] Each of these testimonies normalized the violence of the Ott household and pathologized Anna.

The court issued a summons to Anna via the hospital superintendent and to Aurelia in Chillicothe, but neither woman replied within the required forty days and thus did not testify in any form. No evidence indicates how, when, or if the summons reached Anna. No evidence indicates that the attorney assigned to her spoke with her.

In October 1881 the Dane County Court dissolved the marriage of Anna and George Ott on the basis of Anna's insanity, agreeing that George had neither caused nor contributed to her insanity. While evidence indicates that community knowledge of the violence of the Ott household was widespread and that marital violence eased her diagnosis, in the 1881 divorce her diagnosis of insanity and its consequences had erased such knowledge and blamed her for any lingering stories or allegations. Household violence and its resulting trauma and harm facilitated the insanity diagnosis, but the ableist manner by which the diagnosis rendered Anna unreliable or at blame for the violence then erased or at least blurred the household violence. This suggests that historians of familial violence must pay more attention to medical pathologization and the cultural work that it carries out. Patriarchy and ableism, when working together, reinforced and justified each other. Anna's pathologization by Wisconsin State Hospital physicians and by George himself allowed George to remove himself from the marriage with few economic consequences, an untainted reputation, and the ability to remarry.[113]

The workloads of asylum superintendents likely contributed to the omission of the Ott divorce from Anna's medical file, but the lack of such notations also was due to late nineteenth-century understandings of trauma, psychological disabilities, and their causes. Nineteenth-century physicians generally understood insanity to have organic causes. External life events could serve as kindling to ignite already existing organic defects, but such events likely only built on already existing defects. And apparently the consequences of organic defects varied geographically. Mendota's 1875 annual report stated that the physical causes of insanity "operate with peculiar force in Wisconsin."[114]

In addition to the divorce, events recorded in the economic records of Anna's guardianship files further complicate analyses of Anna, the diagnostic assessment made of her by asylum physicians, and daily life inside late nineteenth-century institutions. For example, throughout 1875 and 1876 the hospital superintendent noted that Anna attacked staff, caused "considerable injury" to others, was at least once placed in the crib, and behaved as "fault finding" and "officious." Also during this time, however, financial records indicate that Madison dressmaker Cecilia Hurley made numerous visits to the hospital in order to properly fit Anna with new clothing. Muslin cloth, embroidery floss, at least six dozen buttons, alpaca, silk yarn, wool, and a new shawl became part of her wardrobe. These two very different kinds of primary sources—reports on Anna's life—paint markedly different and nearly irreconcilable scenes. One source portrays a violent, uncontrolled madwoman, and the other depicts a respectable woman seeking a new wardrobe. Imagining that the woman of the first portrayal held still long enough to be fitted for clothing is difficult.

From March 1877 to April 1879 only four entries totaling twenty-two words appear in Anna's case file. Taken together, the descriptions in the case file—excited, quarrelsome, abusive, delusional, no improvement—paint a dismal picture of ill-being. Economic records, however, once again complicate the picture. During this time Anna received canned and fresh fruit, significant unspecified dry goods, and garlic to season her food. She added a bureau, a washstand, and a rocking chair to her living quarters. Seamstress Hurley spent at least fifteen days at Mendota in 1878 in addition to the sewing work done on Anna's wardrobe while at her own home. Most tantalizing to me is Anna's July 12, 1877, purchase of a $3.50 dictionary. Her personal subscriptions to the local newspaper meant that she did not have to join others in common areas to read the shared newspapers. Perhaps she wrote letters, made notes in a diary, or read novels. Perhaps she simply enjoyed words while she sat in her rocking chair.

In March 1880, the same month that Tredway paid bills for orders of fruit, cologne, and a new dress, Dunning and Sumner, druggists in Madison, delivered a thermometer to the Mendota Asylum "for the use of Mrs. Anna B. Ott."[115] As a biographer, I desperately want this to be a medical thermometer rather than a weather thermometer. Medical clinicians used thermometers in this period in order to diagnose patients. Given Anna's history as a practicing physician, she could have been practicing medicine while a diagnosed madwoman inside the asylum. Hospital superintendents frequently complained about her "impudent" and "faultfinding" nature. Perhaps she disapproved of hospital medical services and took it upon herself to serve as a clinician. Perhaps she bartered her skills to acquire privileges and freedoms or to avoid violence. The only evidence remaining is the receipt for a thermometer from a local druggist, but it is the druggist from which Anna purchased medical supplies prior to her institutionalization.

These details of clothing, furniture, and a dictionary suggest a human being of desires, personality, and interests far beyond Anna's case file. In addition, the details of the case file suggest a human being far beyond her economic records. Taken together, these two markedly different sources suggest that what asylum superintendents considered important, Anna did not. They suggest that the power of superintendents to determine, assess, and even know about a patient's daily life was relatively weak.

This is not to suggest that institutionalization at the Wisconsin State Hospital for the Insane had little impact on Anna's life. Nor does this suggest that she desired her confinement and considered it pleasant. It suggests that despite the incredible authority built into medical case files and the accompanying inferences of diagnoses within them, case files need to be interrogated as primary sources (just as all primary sources need interrogation). Together these sources suggest an ongoing, contentious battle of wills between Anna and asylum staff. The strength of patriarchal ableism coexisted messily alongside Anna's privileges of class and profession. Structural intersectionality coexisted with individual circumstances. While most individuals in hospitals for the insane lacked her specifics, all of them had desires, stories, and resources outside of and in addition to their diagnoses.

7. Anna Ott, Economic Agent

THE WISCONSIN STATE HOSPITAL for the Insane, into which Dr. Anna B. Ott entered, was a significant economic enterprise whose daily workings generated immense income for the local community. Counties and cities fought to have asylums placed near them because of this economic benefit. In 1873, when Anna entered the state hospital, the asylum routinely employed approximately 130 people in both skilled and unskilled positions; 43 of those positions turned over at least once during the year, for a total of at least 173 people employed during the year.[1] In 1884 the then superintendent proudly stated that about 70 percent of people institutionalized at Mendota labored at Mendota, including some of the "most disturbed." While the growing profession of psychiatry always and only referred to inmate labor as a tool in the curative arsenal—alongside drugs and behavioral controls—the unpaid and coerced labor of those considered insane greatly benefited the budgets of institutions such as the Wisconsin State Hospital for the Insane. The institution then benefited the regional economy and its development.

Like the institution as a whole, Anna remained intensely connected to and interwoven with the larger Madison economy. Estimations of the value of her property holdings varied throughout the years of her guardianship but ran from $12,000 to $25,000. (For comparison, $25,000 in 1875 equaled approximately $600,000 in 2018.)[2] Her guardian, William Tredway, documented receipt of payments from those who used her rental properties and from those for whom she had provided mortgages. He paid taxes on her properties and investments. In the first year or two he expressed his great frustration at the dismal state of her financial record-keeping, the bills left unpaid, and her failure to pay taxes in previous years. He made quarterly payments for Anna's care. He managed the day-to-day details of the care and management of her properties, which were immense. Such details included, for example, paying $9.00 for roof repair in 1875, $2.50 for the privy to be cleaned out in 1877, and $6.30 for sidewalk repairs in 1880.[3] Significant and specific documentation remains regarding the management of Anna's property, financial resources, and investments.

The bulk of Tredway's financial documentation, however, pertains to Anna's spending. During her years of institutionalization, Anna spent money, and she did so to make her life tolerable. Though Anna's medical records make clear that hospital staff sometimes moved her from ward to ward, Anna augmented her living quarters with her own furniture. In December 1874 Tredway paid nine dollars for a washstand, delivered to Anna at the hospital.[4] In August 1877 she bought a dressing bureau, in 1878 a rocking chair, and in 1881 a bamboo chair.[5] Anna subscribed to the local newspaper. She enjoyed boat rides on Lake Mendota.[6] She ordered and received her own tableware, including china and tea sets.[7] She had perfume, soap, hairbrushes, hosiery, and handkerchiefs delivered.[8]

Clothing and food constituted the majority of Anna's spending from the time she entered Mendota in 1872 until 1885.[9] During this time seamstresses regularly (sometimes every quarter) visited her in order to create new clothing. For example, in April 1874 seamstress Henrietta Hopkins made Anna a dress of black silk with trimmings in addition to socks and shoes.[10] A December 1876 bill included five dozen buttons ($1.92) and forty-six yards of alpaca (likely woven cloth, $50.24)—perhaps for blankets, socks, or a coat.[11] In February 1881 Tredway paid the $5.62 bill of a local seamstress who had spent four and a half days, part of them with Anna at the hospital, constructing and fitting several dresses.[12]

Anna also spent money on food, largely fresh fruit but also canned fruit during the months it was out of season in Wisconsin. For example, in March 1880 Tredway received a local grocer's bill for six cases of pears (thirty-five cans in each case), six cases of peaches (thirty-five each), two cases of grapes, and two cases of plums.[13] Similarly, in January 1883 Tredway paid a bill for three cans each of peaches, pears, and apricots; a can each of grapes, gum drops, and egg plums; a dozen oranges; half a dozen lemons; and two dozen dates.[14] Businesses sent bills to Tredway after numerous purchases added up.

Thus, even while an asylum inmate, Anna remained an important community consumer of benefit to a sizable number of local businesses. While the quantity and luxurious nature of her purchases were unique, the importing of goods into the asylum was not. In 1873, for example, the family of asylum inmate Alice Howard sent her a dress, two undergarments, two pairs of

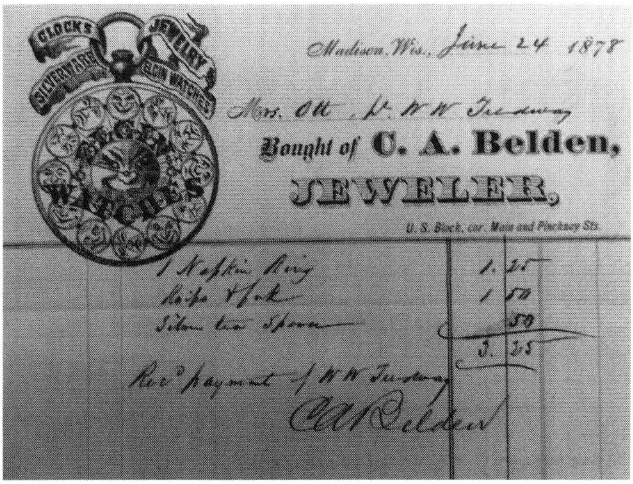

Image 6. A June 1878 receipt for a napkin ring, a knife and fork, and a silver tea spoon totaling $3.25 from C. A. Belden, Jeweler, in Madison, Wisconsin. Ott Guardianship Files.

stockings, a pair of slippers, and a hat.[15] Families and individuals frequently sent material goods into the asylum.

Anna was not alone among institutionalized people who continued their engagement in economic production outside of the asylum. Anna's fellow resident and fellow legal incompetent Anders Hedman, for example, spent approximately eight months of every year at the State Hospital for the Insane and joined his mother for four months every summer in order to work the family farm.[16] He did this for twenty-two years, from 1876 to 1898. Perhaps his family begged the asylum superintendent for his labor due to their economic necessity, or perhaps Hedman eloped (the period term for running away). Perhaps the coming of spring and extended daylight hours loosened Hedman's impairments, which once again settled in with the shortening of the days. Whatever the reason, he went to the family farm every summer to labor, and his family depended on his labor. Similarly, institutionalized mothers left documentation of sewing clothing for their children, which they then sent home for daily usage. They did their own household labor while still institutionalized as insane.[17] Asylum residents such as these mothers, Hedman, and Anna remained integrally connected to and engaged with the larger community's labor and economic systems. Some families did and could remain dependent on the labor of those in asylums.

In addition, the economies inside the asylum were highly tied to and interwoven with economic systems outside the asylum. Goods and cash moved constantly back and forth, and local businesses benefited immensely. In 1873, for example, the asylum provided cash for labor and/or goods to approximately 210 businesses and individuals outside the asylum. The asylum hired skilled and unskilled laborers for short-term specific tasks such as repairing masonry work on the front steps, transporting an inmate to another institution, and building a new smokestack. The asylum also purchased material goods of which it had need or of which it had not produced an adequate supply, including crockery for the kitchen, ice, and liquor. In 1873 this totaled $119,296.65.[18] Asylums served as medicalized sites of capitalism.

Historians have long known that asylum inmates engaged in economic production while institutionalized. Inmates were assigned and sometimes forced to labor. Nineteenth-century asylum physician-superintendents espoused labor as an essential part of the cure process that would return one to self-management. For example, Dr. D. F. Boughton, one of the first superintendents of the Wisconsin State Hospital for the Insane, called inmate labor "a powerful curative means." Physicians argued that labor resulted in exercise, self-worth, social worth, and mental focus, all believed to contribute to curing those diagnosed as insane. Asylum personnel interpreted a refusal to labor as a refusal to cooperate with medical treatment and worthy of punishment. Conveniently, of course, inmate labor greatly reduced the expenses of the institution and frequently generated income for the asylum. Dr. Boughton may have considered inmate labor "a powerful curative," but he also sought to use it to improve the physical grounds and economy of the asylum.[19]

The forced production of goods such as those listed below, in addition to tasks such as cooking or cleaning, reduced hospital expenses immensely. For example, the sewing room at the Wisconsin State Hospital included one paid seamstress, who labored with "considerable help" from female residents. In 1873 the curative labor of this group of women produced an immense amount of goods, which greatly reduced asylum costs. Asylum women produced 2,212 pieces of clothing and home goods (see table 2). The cleaning, cooking, and laundry labor done by female asylum inmates often remained invisible economically, just as it did in individual households. Approximately thirty "female patients from the different wards" turned the seven hundred bushels of potatoes grown by male residents, along with other farm goods such as hogs, pork, and milk, into meals for over six hundred people.[20] Because such labor did not generate goods that could be sold or tabulated, inmates' hours tended not to be included in yearly asylum reports. The erasure of women's labor in both the private sphere and the public sphere of the asylum was linked.

Table 2. Wisconsin State Hospital for the Insane Clothing and Bedding Production, 1873

Product	Quantity	Product	Quantity
Dresses	243	Straw ticks	51
Shirts	165	Towels	488
Chemise	100	Roller towels	37
Drawers	119	Sun bonnets	78
Nightgowns	134	Suspender pairs	172
Skirts	60	Aprons	8
Mittens	106	Waterproof capes	25
Camisoles	10	Waterproof cloaks	1
Sheets	247	Handkerchiefs	168

Source: Data derived from the *Annual Report of the Board of Trustees of the Wisconsin State Hospital for the Insane for the Year Ending September 30, 1873* (Madison: James Ross, State Printer, 1873).

The farm grounds of the Wisconsin State Hospital for the Insane were sites of immensely economically productive and time-consuming male labor. The grains, fruits, vegetables, and animals of the hospital farm fed its inmates, generated income when surplus goods were sold, and, like the household goods produced by women, greatly reduced institutional expenditures. The 1873 production of eight hundred bushels of beets and four tons of winter squash, just to isolate two examples, would feed many people. Both could be sweetened by the 128 gallons of maple syrup (one gallon of maple syrup requires 30–50 gallons of sap) generated that year (see table 3).

Attendants and physicians assigned residents to labor believed appropriate for an individual's sex, race, and class. Men tended to be assigned farm or industrial-type labor. Women labored in the smaller gardens, kitchen, laundry, and sewing shop; they also cleaned the buildings and raised chickens. While no evidence exists of a racial division of labor at the Wisconsin State Hospital for the Insane, the number of African American and Native residents remained incredibly small. One can presume that they received the dirtiest or most unappealing jobs (e.g., shoveling manure, removing human waste, boiling laundry). For institutionalized members of the upper class, such as Anna Ott, appropriate labor meant no recognized labor. Indeed, at one point a physician made a note in her medical record that she "remains idle," indicating not a value judgment but that she did not labor.[21] Labor hierarchies inside the asylum thus replicated those outside the asylum.

Compulsory labor runs throughout US history. Like insane asylums, prisons often required labor of their inmates but defined it as punishment and,

Table 3. Wisconsin State Hospital for the Insane Agricultural Production, 1873

Product	Quantity	Product	Quantity
Wheat	404 bushels	Clover seed	10 bushels
Oats	1910 bushels	Green peas	12 bushels
Corn, field (for animals)	1499 bushels	Onions	200 bushels
Corn, sweet (for humans)	74 bushels	Early turnips	100 bushels
Potatoes	700 bushels	Grapes	200 pounds
Carrots	500 bushels	Cabbage heads	2,000
Beets	800 bushels	Winter squash	4 tons
Tomatoes	100 bushels	Summer squash	2 tons
Apples	75 bushels	Hay	150 tons
Strawberries	7 bushels	Straw	75 tons
Timothy seed	6 bushels	Corn stalks	40 tons
Pork, live weight	13,600 pounds	Chickens	75
Stock hogs	2,500 pounds	Milk	9,153 gallons
Beef, live weight	6,500 pounds	Beans	20 bushels
Veal	800 pounds	Maple syrup	128 gallons
Turkeys	18		

Note: A U.S. bushel equals 35.2 liters or 8 gallons.
Source: Data derived from the *Annual Report of the Board of Trustees of the Wisconsin State Hospital for the Insane for the Year Ending September 30, 1873* (Madison: James Ross, State Printer, 1873).

sometimes, as rehabilitation (an "honest" labor). Poor farms often required labor and assigned it in gender and racially specific ways, but they explained labor as the necessary contribution of charity recipients. Racism defined enslaved people as incapable of self-management; thus, compulsory labor was a necessity. The labor of insane asylum inmates is unique in its prescriptive and curative nature because it was undergirded by the hope of restoring self-management. The coerced labor of asylum inmates served to strengthen capitalism and help emergent state-building. Its prescriptive nature hid its fundamentally capitalist and laboring characteristics.

Guardian William Tredway never exercised control over Anna's spending, despite the incredibly large quantity of food, furniture, seamstress supplies, reading goods, and other material supplies she ordered delivered to the Mendota Insane Asylum. He never exercised control despite his legal right to do so and his legal obligation to insure that money was not squandered. He simply signed approval and paid the bills over and over and over again—highly unusual behavior for a guardian.

It is important to acknowledge that while the receipts for purchases made between 1873 and 1893 pile up, there is no specific evidence that Anna actually received the purchased goods herself. In 1880 the Wisconsin state legislature created a special committee to investigate the affairs of the Wisconsin State Hospital for the Insane. Their report determined that "patients" were "humanely treated and properly clothed," though it suggested more nursing staff and advised that the "serving of hash for breakfast every day in the year should cease." Most important to state officials, however, the committee found the hospital's financial records to be a mess. They considered the annual printed reports to be "entirely unreliable" due not to fraud but to the "exceedingly confused condition of the accounts." The committee criticized the superintendent (Dr. D. F. Boughton) for "the habit of borrowing large sums of money from his employees."[22] If some of Anna's funds or goods were filtered into the pockets of others, it may not have been discernible. And as discussed earlier, theft remained highly possible. However, given the diligence of Anna's guardian, William Tredway, the respect he received from members of the Madison community, and his prior management of huge Civil War budgets, it is unlikely that such theft happened in large amounts.

Tredway chose not to curtail or control Anna's spending, but he was not a pushover. What does Tredway's clear avoidance of exercising control mean?

On an immediate and practical level, my analysis is that the court assigned Tredway as a means of hedging its bets. The judge who appointed him had undoubtedly been included in many a dinner or barroom conversation about the volatile Ott marriage. The assignment of Tredway expressed the court's disapproval of George's violence, but the slap on his hand was accompanied by the institutionalization of Anna and the court's determination of her incompetency. The court and the community generally remained highly suspicious of Anna and her behaviors, but they did not want to reward George. Local businesses wanted Anna to continue to spend. Tredway simply paid the bills.

Anna's privileges of class and profession, even while she was institutionalized, add complexity to the frequent accusations by asylum personnel that she was officious and imperious. As diagnostic terms, "officious" and "imperious" are deeply gendered and judgmental. Anna was a shrewd businesswoman who had left her first marriage with significant funds. She had invested those funds wisely and likely held a greater net worth than nearly all asylum staff combined at the time of her institutionalization. She understood herself to be a physician of knowledge and experience who was capable of assessing the diagnostic skills and actions of those who ran the asylum. Clothing, furniture, food, and other material goods signified power. She could have used fruits and vegetables as a form of currency within the institution. (One wonders how quickly she could have eaten a case of canned fruit.) Undoubtedly, she was officious and imperious. As one physician complained at the time of her

1881 divorce, her guardian allowed her to have "everything that was suitable and even more than was necessary for her comfort."[23]

In his 1874 report to the board of trustees of the Wisconsin State Hospital, Superintendent Mark Ranney noted that many hospital residents "become attached to their single room." When that was the case they often "decorate it with pictures, flowers or autumn leaves, or articles of their own handwork, and altogether feel a home interest in it." As a physician, he argued that "this state of feeling is always desirable, and should always be cultivated."[24] Anna's purchases, however, went far beyond what Ranney thought was therapeutic.

On a theoretical and analytical level, Anna's ability to access and benefit from her financial resources matters—and messes up my tidy analytical frameworks. In the constricted and miserable context of the asylum, and in the constricted and miserable context of patriarchal ableism, financial resources provided a means for Anna to exert will and agency. Her resources and her access to them improved her daily life in substantial ways. The interlocking web of structural forces that encircled Anna, the Wisconsin State Hospital for the Insane, and the Dane County Circuit Court had strength and was real but those forces do not overlie neatly all the details of individual lives. Put bluntly, patriarchy and ableism permeated everything, but at the same time, George and members of the local legal system cannot be dismissed solely as evil men who locked Anna away to get at her property. Analysis—and life—are messy and not that simple.

Anna's daughter, Aurelia, left evidence of continued contact with her mother. In November 1873 Aurelia asked for some of Anna's money to pay for a visit, but both her stepfather, George, and Tredway refused. George expressed hope to Superintendent Ranney that Anna "will be getting more reasonable." Aurelia again wrote seeking news of her mother in the fall of 1874 and the summer of 1876. By 1876 Aurelia had divorced her husband, Dayton Morgan, and lived in Chillicothe near her father, Dr. Jonathan Miesse.[25] Aurelia visited her mother in the fall of 1879, staying for about a month in Madison. She reported a "pleasant visit" with her mother but was called back to Chillicothe earlier than planned. Her father was "dangerously ill," and she was "needed at the bedside." We only know of this visit because during her time in Madison Aurelia was robbed of all her cash by a pickpocket and had to borrow money from Tredway, who noted the event.[26] It is probable that Aurelia visited her mother at other times unmarked by theft. Sometime around 1890 Aurelia married again and moved to Jacksonville, Florida, which made for a much more onerous and expensive journey to Madison, Wisconsin.

Many of the families of those institutionalized at the Wisconsin State Hospital for the Insane sought sustained contact with either their family member or hospital staff, just as Aurelia did. Each month the hospital superintendent received over fifty letters, frequently as many as one hundred, from family members expressing concern, fears, and hopes and sharing news. The impact of diagnosis and prescriptive institutionalization reached far beyond the institution and far beyond the individual.

Letters frequently focused on what to do if a family member died while institutionalized at Mendota or whether or not a family member still lived. Transporting a body home could be expensive, as could a burial, and doing so in hot Wisconsin summers was difficult regardless of one's income. Communicating could be difficult, especially if family members were illiterate. An 1873 telegram simply stated, "Is my wife dead answer."[27] Upon receiving notice that her husband was "feeble," Mrs. Cyrene Green requested that if he was "taken away," he would be buried at the hospital.[28] D. A. Davis asked that the grave of his daughter be marked with "the day of the month and her name" so that he could later recover her remains.[29] Some asked that their family member's remains be sent home via train or carriage.[30]

Many family members wrote to the hospital superintendent rather than to their institutionalized loved one to share family news. It is likely that many institutionalized people were not allowed mail, a common practice across the country at insane asylums. Marie Allen sadly sent news to her husband of the death "of our little girl" via the superintendent and asked, "Please inform me just how he [her husband] rcvd" the news. Louis Blank asked that the superintendent tell his wife that their seven-year-old son was dying: "I have no hope to save him." Edward Bishop, who wrote regularly to Superintendent Ranney seeking information about his wife, asked that Ranney share information about the children. "The baby is with Mrs. Paice," he wrote, "and the two oldest is with Edward Connars."[31]

Many of the letter writers expressed great love and pain, particularly those who desperately sought information about the family member and whether or not the family member spoke of them. Edgar Ray asked about his wife: "Does she inquire of hir baby tell hir it is well and if she comes to hir rite mind tell hir that hir Baby is at my folks."[32] Elisa Bright wrote that she had "such an intense longing" to learn of her sister that she was "almost distracted with anxiety about her."[33] Dora Servis was "deeply concerned" about Mrs. Barr and her unhappiness: "Is she restless; does she act like she was unhappy and did not want to stay there; does she walk out and notice the beauty of the flowers or the green foliage."[34] S. S. Luscombe begged for news, stating that such would enable him "to pass the weary days and sleepless nights more comfortably." He sent fruit and letters from his children to their mother.[35] Other families sent clothing, even when they could not afford it.[36] Miss L.

M. Williams wanted to make sure that her father got the violin she had sent and asked that he be told that "we are living at Grandpa's this winter."[37]

Some family members feared what would happen if their family member came home again and wrote asking hospital staff to do what they could to detain the family member. Emily Sandford had received threatening letters from her husband and asked hospital staff to "see that he don't get away, for we are not safe here with him." She lived "in fear that he will run off and come home again."[38] William Eckels had escaped twice and "made his family a great deal of trouble while at home." His wife asked a local official to write "and see that he don't get away."[39] Some families wrote of formerly institutionalized family members they sought to send back, generally due to violence.[40] One family sought Dr. Ranney's assistance after their family member had returned home, only to pawn everything in the house, including the clothes he wore, to buy liquor.[41] Peter Kavenaugh's brother was causing no problems, but he had shown up at home after escaping from the hospital, and the family did not know what to do.[42]

These letters document sharply the transition from family care to institutional care, hastened by the Civil War and postwar institutional developments. Prior to the Civil War, few US residents ever entered any kind of hospital or institution. Between 1830 and the 1890s, the number of state and private institutions grew exponentially. This written and economic evidence reveals that families continued to expect, seek, and create connections with their loved ones despite their removal from the family setting and a growing reliance on institutions.

In 1893, the year that Anna died, J. B. Andrews, president of the American Medico-Psychological Association, addressed his society's members about their noble cause. He urged them to remember the immense medical progress made in their profession, which had "added immeasurably to the comfort of their inmates." "All the institutions," he went on, whether called asylum or hospital, "are conducted as places for the care and cure of the sick, rather than for mere retention of the insane."[43] Andrews and his medical counterparts across the nation, as well as the numerous state legislators who voted to fund the ever-growing number of state institutions, understood their purpose and focus to be medical.

The breadth and reach of asylums, however, went far beyond medicine. Anna Ott knew herself to be medically diagnosed and prescriptively institutionalized at the Wisconsin State Hospital for the Insane. There is no doubt that she and the hundreds of other institutionalized people she encountered over her twenty years in Mendota, as well as the hundreds of thousands across the country, experienced their institutionalization to be far more than medical. Families and individuals experienced institutionalization as a complex and ongoing medical, legal, and economic process. The details of the impact of the combined forces of medicine, law, and economics varied somewhat by race and class, but the power of this trio, as well as their inseparability, did not. In addition, geographic communities experienced the development of institutions medically, legally, and economically. As this chapter has shown, nineteenth-century insane asylums altered communities. They became huge economic markets, provided goods to the local economy, created employment opportunities and also provided laborers, generated a demand for attorneys and new legal processes, and medicalized behaviors sometimes not previously considered pathological. The reach of nineteenth-century asylums extended far beyond their geographical boundaries, their influence on individuals, families, and communities buttressed by the entwined structures, ideologies, and practices of medicine, law, and economics.

8. Remembering Anna Ott

DR. ANNA B. OTT died in 1893 after twenty years in the Wisconsin State Hospital for the Insane, isolated from family and friends and generally erased. Her spending had diminished in 1885. So also did the complaints about her made by medical staff. In 1885, at sixty-six years old, she experienced what the superintendent called a stroke, followed several months later by additional strokes. Tredway resigned as guardian in January 1886. Between 1886 and 1893 several local men served as guardians. Nearly a century and a quarter later, I first struggled to find the nearly unmarked cemetery and then spent almost three hours searching for her grave marker. The Mendota Memorial Cemetery, its current name, is roughly the size of two city lots and contains the bodies of 771 men and women who died while institutionalized at the Wisconsin State Hospital for the Insane. As is the case at nearly all insane asylum cemeteries across the United States, only a handful of those buried at the Mendota Memorial Cemetery have grave markers. The estate of Anna B. Ott paid for the simple flat marker noting her gravesite, a marker easily overgrown by grass and weeds. The rest of the dead lie unnamed and largely unclaimed. The disregard with which they had been treated in death reveals much about their lives and their institutionalization.

Death was a routine part of nineteenth-century institutional life. Anna was one of thirty-nine who died at the Wisconsin State Hospital for the Insane in 1893; in 1894, fifty-one inmates died (an institutional record).[1] Though death was routine, family members frequently struggled to learn news of their institutionalized loved ones. Communication between asylum personnel and family members could be difficult, laborious, and expensive in late nineteenth-century Wisconsin, particularly in winter. The same was true for the transportation of bodies. In 1874 a Mr. Pahl sought news of his wife, Henriette Pahl, for the anxious husband had "heard she lately died there" and wanted to know "if it is so." She had not.[2] Similarly, a friend of a Mr. Stanton wrote in 1876 seeking information: "A rumor is current on the streets that Mrs. Stanton is dead and buried. Mr. Stanton is very anxious to know the truth of it."[3]

Like Mr. Stanton, I am very anxious to know the truth of Dr. Anna B. Ott's death, but as a historical subject she is elusive. Her grave marker conveys the location of her burial and the date of her death but indicates nothing about how she died, if anyone mourned her, or her thoughts and actions during her last days. I do not know if Aurelia knew of her mother's death before her burial, or if the daughter later visited her mother's gravesite. Whether or not any extended family members cared about her death is unknown. Her grave marker is unadorned and uninformative.

Death, however, did not end Anna Ott's story. Over a year after her death she once again hit the national news. Anna, unnamed asylum employees claimed, had issued a dramatic deathbed confession to an unsolved 1857 robbery of the local Wells Fargo office. According to the reported confession, she had robbed a Wells Fargo employee of his key after delivering his wife of a baby, sneaked into the office, and emptied the safe of $8,500. News articles noted that she was a woman of means who built a luxurious home soon after the robbery.[4] These accusations suggested that she accumulated at least some of her wealth via theft, that guile due to either selfishness or insanity drove her actions.

How did *this* become the story? Could the asylum staff see no other reason for the personal wealth of the woman they had dismissed as insane for over twenty years? Did any of them know of her prior life and her guardian's management of her personal property? Anna's diagnosis of insanity became its own story, which retroactively recast everything in her life, even her life story prior to diagnosis. The story of the robbery is tantalizing but unlikely. Anna's numerous strokes, the resulting paralysis, and her confinement to bed raise significant questions about her ability to make such a confession. Her diagnosis told a story about her that was more all-encompassing, explicable, and convenient than logical. Not only were her professional standing and financial skills erased, but their fruits became fruits of criminal insanity.

But even then, the story was not over. A 1930s book of Madison's beautiful homes included the former Ott home built in 1860 by architect August Kutzboch and noted one unique element: each room had two doorways, even the wine cellar. The reason given was that George Ott had feared the violence of his insane wife, Anna, and thus insisted that the architect include two doors in every room so that George could escape from his crazy wife.[5]

How did *this* become the story? In my reading of the evidence, Anna's neighbors, the local alderman, and even the courts believed her allegations of George's violence, even though their efforts to stop it were limited. However, between her last attempt to divorce George in 1870 and the publication of the coffee-table book in the 1930s, George had divorced her, she had spent twenty years in an insane asylum, and she had appeared in newspapers as a bank robber. By 1930 she had become an entertaining town lunatic of community memory. Once again, the diagnosis physicians conferred upon her and the resulting decades of prescriptive institutionalization rewrote Anna's story and then expanded outward to rewrite George's story and that of their home. The violence of the ableist disregard and dismissal of those diagnosed as insane engulfed and then erased the complexities of her life, causing the majority of others to view her as a one-dimensional madwoman. Ableism infused spaces not explicitly medical.

Then there is the story that does not exist. Though Dr. Ott's death was noted briefly in a publication for regional physicians, she is never mentioned in any history of Wisconsin physicians or of female physicians nationally. I have been unable to find evidence that local Madison suffragists or other female physicians supported Anna throughout her years in Wisconsin. Suffragists and other advocates of women's property and marital reform laws supported Elizabeth Packard's efforts to limit the ability of husbands to institutionalize their wives, but none appear to have made note of Anna's situation. Other female physicians supported one another professionally and personally, but Anna remained separated from those networks. While the reasons for this are likely complicated, the ableism of diagnosis once again may be at the core of the issue. Suffragists sought to establish themselves as competent citizens. White suffragists in particular contrasted their respectable and reliable nature with the undesirables—male drunkards, the insane, the criminal, and, in some cases, immigrants and men of color.[6] Anna joined the suffrage campaign relatively early, before it became widely respectable. She then entered the insane asylum just months after attempting to vote. Her sometimes disreputable behavior, coupled with her diagnosis and institutionalization, may have rendered her a distasteful cause to suffragists and female physicians eager to claim respectability.

Distorted through a messy array of historical forces that included ableism, patriarchy, and institutionalization, the life story of Dr. Anna B. Ott was and is shifting terrain. The justifying logic imbedded in her diagnosis and prescriptive institutionalization (re)wrote her life story—her past, her future, and how she would be remembered. Diagnosis served as a reductive gesture, placing her on the "trajectory of that ineluctable narrative" and reducing her story to that of a madwoman whose madness explained everything.[7] Historian Ava Chamberlain found diagnosis to have a similar result in the life story of Elizabeth Tuttle, a woman diagnosed long after her death as the "crazy grandmother" of Puritan theologian Jonathan Edwards.[8] In the words of scholar Elizabeth Lunbeck, diagnoses "acted as templates for life stories . . . filling in what was hidden in those stories' pasts, and, more importantly, endowing them with a future"—or, in this case, a lack thereof.[9] Diagnoses' supposed scientific and thus value-free neutrality erased or made invisible even the possibility that politics, power, money, or gender hierarchies might influence perceptions of Anna's behaviors, success, and riches.[10] An insanity diagnosis made the later stories of a bank robbery and architectural oddities possible and erased stories of Anna's professional career, activism, and financial gain. Receiving a diagnosis meant that Anna could no longer be the diagnostic physician herself but only receive the diagnostic expertise of others. For her, diagnosis resulted in containment and trauma. The ableism undergirding Anna's insanity diagnosis permeated legal, familial, and activist contexts both outside and inside the walls of medicine in the late nineteenth-century United States.

Thus, Anna Barbara Blaser Miesse Ott easily slipped into historical oblivion—the teenage immigrant who traversed the Atlantic, the Ohio physician's wife, the female physician of Madison, the survivor of turbulent marriages, and the Sixth Ward manic.

The elephant in the room is the question of Anna Ott's madness. Was she insane? I argue against this question. First, there is the issue of historical change. The criteria for a psychiatric diagnosis have changed dramatically between 1873 and today. This leaves me as a historian wondering whether to use an 1873 or an 1893 physician's manual, the 1952 edition of the *Diagnostic and Statistical Manual of Mental Disorders* (*DSM*), or the *DSM* II, III, IV, or V (2013). Even more profound and substantive than historical change, however, is that, as medical historians have long recognized, diagnoses are historically situated expressions of cultural values that do cultural work. Questions about the accuracy of Anna's diagnosis replicate the power structures and assumptions that justified her institutionalization and illegitimization. Questions about diagnostic accuracy reveal nothing about the breadth of diagnostic labels, the messy historical forces that strengthen and justify diagnoses, and the messy ways that diagnoses strengthen and justify historical forces such as patriarchy and ableism. Nor do these questions reveal anything about the interests of those with the power to issue diagnoses. In other words, the room, to massively paraphrase Virginia Woolf, was never one of Anna Ott's own. A diagnosis of mania enabled others to act upon her in messy ways inclusive of but reaching beyond patriarchy and ableism. Diagnosis was someone else writing the story, narrativizing upon her. And throughout that story, Anna Ott resisted.

Anna Ott lived a life sometimes difficult, sometimes traumatic, and sometimes privileged. The "accuracy" of her diagnosis, from the vantage point of over a century later, does not change her lived experience.

This is not an argument that psychiatric disabilities do not exist. Indeed, psychiatric disabilities, sometimes resisted and sometimes claimed, have existed in numerous historical and cultural contexts. However, and this is what I seek to argue, what it has meant to be insane and the definitions of insanity (as well as sanity, health, and illness) have changed immensely throughout history. This has to be forefronted. When applying contemporary psychological insights, definitions, and analyses to the past, we must avoid ahistoricism. We cannot ignore the fact that, historically, structures of power such as race, class, gender, sexual ideals, religiosity, ideas about the normative body, conquest, and colonialism have profoundly influenced definitions of madness (insanity, mental illness). Power structures have shaped who gets to be the diagnoser. In addition, those in power have often used definitions of mental illness to maintain their power.

Perhaps a productive way to reframe questions about the accuracy of Anna's diagnosis is to consider instead the human and scholarly desire to impose neatness. Historian Susan Cahn has suggested that feminist disability history can help unpack "both the 'biography' of an illness and the biographies of people said to suffer from it."[11] The example of Anna is a reminder that the history of insanity and those diagnosed with it is profoundly entangled with other historical factors, including money, patriarchy, familial violence, and the institutions of state-building. Her life is a forceful reminder that a stigmatized diagnosis has powerful consequences and that those consequences reach far beyond medical frameworks into communities, social structures, and individual biographies. Her life also reminds me that patriarchy and ableism, while strong, are never all-powerful. While frameworks of analysis are vital and must be intersectional in nature, they rarely if ever map tidily onto individual human lives. We as scholars need to continue to foster analytical tools and practices to robustly and messily analyze messy histories.

Biography is a powerful and effective tool. The strength and richness of biography is that, when done well, biographies forefront lived experiences while simultaneously embedding those lived experiences in large-scale social and historical structures. In the case of Anna B. Ott, a biography enables an analysis of how ableism and patriarchy intersected, along with varying other systems, to impact an individual life. Strong biographies are inherently intersectional. I intend *Money, Marriage, and Madness* to make clear how understanding human lives, past and present, individual and corporate, requires analytical use of both structural forces and individual circumstances.

Despite these strengths, academic historians tend to reside uneasily with biographies. In a 2009 *American Historical Review* roundtable, David Nasaw described biography as the "profession's unloved stepchild, occasionally but grudgingly let in the door, more often shut outside with the riffraff." Lois Banner similarly noted that historians "often rank biography as an inferior type of history."[12] I encourage historians to shake off any reluctance or shame they may feel about writing biography and embrace the unique potential biographies contain for deepening (and sometimes altering) historical understandings both structural and focused. Biographical examinations of those who have been erased, in this case, a woman diagnosed as insane, have potential to be radical sites of rich and intersectional learning.[13]

Biographies are sites of potential theoretical advancement when they blend analyses of social systems with considerations of daily life. For example, an intersectional and messy analysis of Anna Ott's life provides a means to respond to calls from feminist disability studies scholars for rigorous attention to mental disability and bodymindedness.[14] Anna, however, is neither the madwoman in the attic, the homeless lunatic on the streets, the emerging feminist locked amid disturbing yellow wallpaper, nor the woman who turned to madness as a form of feminist resistance. She is neither glamorous, heroic, nor a metaphor.[15] Like the life stories of so many other disabled people, particularly those considered insane and female, Anna's life story became a chimera used to strengthen the ableist boundaries between sanity and insanity, to bulwark patriarchy, and to legitimate institutionalization. Her life reveals the immense strength, breadth, and impact of ableism, as well as the impossibility of detangling ableism from patriarchy, class differentials, and the institutions and processes of state-building. Her life also, however, reveals the weakness of structural forces and the ways by which individuals undermined and contradicted them. Good history requires messy analyses.

It is tempting to use what are ultimately empty archetypes to characterize Anna Barbara Blaiser Miesse Ott: a victim of marital and institutional patriarchy, a feminist heroine of resistance and valor, a confidence woman or con artist whose luck finally ran out, or a lunatic who tainted all she touched. I think, however, that the most honest of characterizations, the one most true to the paucity of primary sources from which to tell the story, is that Anna simply did the best she could to change her complicated life circumstances amid an interlocking and competing array of social institutions.

Notes

Introduction

1. For explanations of bodymind and the ways by which it is used to understand the body and mind as a single, integrated unit, see Price, "The Bodymind Problem"; and Carter, "Teaching with Trauma."

2. Metzl, *The Protest Psychosis*; Epstein, *Inclusion*; Reverby, "Inclusion and Exclusion"; Burch and Joyner, *Unspeakable*; Metzl and Kirkland, *Against Health.*

3. Clare, *Brilliant Imperfection*, 42.

4. Goffman, *Asylums*; Foucault, *Madness and Civilization*; Rothman, *The Discovery*; Rothman, *Conscience and Convenience*; Grob, *Mental Institutions*; Grob, *Mental Illness*; Szasz, *The Myth*; Tomes, *A Generous Confidence*; Dwyer, *Homes for the Mad*; Lunbeck, *The Psychiatric Persuasion*; Reaume, *Remembrance of Patients Past*; Reiss, *Theaters of Madness.* Kathleen M. Brian provides a brief but strong analysis of this historiography in "'The Weight.'"

5. Examples of this include Penney and Stastny, *The Lives*; Metzl, *The Protest Psychosis*; Burch and Joyner, *Unspeakable.*

6. Goodley, *Dis/Ability Studies*, 32.

7. For more on messiness, see Nielsen, "Dr. Anna B. Ott."

8. Hartman, "Venus in Two Acts," 11.

9. Foucault, "Lives of Infamous Men," 162.

10. As will be seen, Ott has no direct living descendants whom I could consult regarding this decision.

Chapter 1. Mrs. Anna Miesse, Local Doctor's Wife

1. Hartog, *Man and Wife*, 101–2.

2. Sklar, *Catharine Beecher*, 151.

3. Beecher, *A Treatise*, 44.

4. Heilbrun, *Writing*, 37.

5. Records from Ott's second marriage also provide false information about her medical education. Whether or not this information is accurate is completely unknown to me.

6. Ulrich Blaser (1795–1872) married Anna Barbara Leeman, who used the name Barbara (1796–1863), in 1817. They arrived in New York on July 31, 1834, with Jann/John (1817–), Anna Barbara Blaser (1819–93), Friedrich/Frederick (1821–63), Christian (1823–70), Anna Elizabeth, who used the name Elizabeth (1824–95), Gottlieb (1826–58), Maria/Mary (1828–), Sophia (1831–55), Godfrey (1833–1914), Ferdinand (about 1836–), and William (about 1841–). There may have been an Elizabeth born approximately 1829, Caroline approximately 1838, Therisa approximately 1839, and a child stillborn approximately 1840.

7. "Benjamin Franklin Miesse," in *Portrait and Biographical Record*, 136–37; "Dr. Jonathan Miesse," in *History of Ross*, 218.

8. This detail is based on the marriage date and information about Cornelius in the 1856 divorce case filed by Jonathan Miesse against Anna (a case later withdrawn).

9. 1840 US Census, Adelphia, Ohio. Adelphia was geographically closer to Jonathan's brothers than Anna's family. In 1840 area census takers only took note of heads of household, but presumably Anna and Cornelius resided with Jonathan.

10. Brown, "Chillicothe's Elite."

11. Rippley, "The Chillicothe Germans," 212.

12. Ibid., 215.

13. Ibid., 217.

14. See the 1930 placard on the Zion Reformed Church of Chillicothe, Ohio, http://www.waymarking.com/waymarks/WMCoET_Zion_Reformed_Church__Winesburg_OH, accessed February 5, 2017.

15. Rowe, "In Strength & Struggle"; Salafia, *Slavery's Borderland*, 166.

16. Stephen Middleton quoted in Salafia, *Slavery's Borderland*, 152.

17. Thanks to the staff of E. M. Smith Jewelers for letting me visit the home, which is now a private business.

18. "Dr. Jonathan Miesse," in *History of Ross*, 218. Jonathan's brother Gabriel's medical education had purportedly "begun when he was a mere child and was conducted chiefly under the direct superintendence of a private teacher, Dr. Charles Quinedon, a finely cultured physician from Prussia." The same may have been true for Jonathan. See *A Biographical History*.

19. Shryock, *Medical Licensing*, 23: "In some cases, state examining boards were created. In other instances, state medical societies were granted power to test and license, and this might be done by one central board or by censors chosen for particular counties or districts. The testing was done largely if not exclusively by medical men, usually in the form of oral quizzes which must have differed from state to state, or county to county." See also Wendler, "Doctors and Diseases," 231.

20. Like his brothers Jonathan and Benjamin, the oldest Miesse brother, Gabriel LaFayette, attended medical school during the 1845–46 year, but he instead chose

to attend the Eclectic Medical Institute in Cincinnati. See http://brianaltonenmph.com/6-history-of-medicine-and-pharmacy/eclectic-medicine-eclectics-1845–1875/ accessed February 5, 2017.

21. Abrahams, *Extinct Medical Schools*, chap. 1; Norwood, *Medical Education*, 94–97.

22. *Public Ledger* (Philadelphia), March 5, 1846, 2; "Valedictory Address of the Graduating Class, Medical Department of Pennsylvania College for the Session of 1845–1846," D. Gilbert, M.D. (Philadelphia: King and Baird Printers, 1846).

23. This detail is based on the marriage date and information about Cornelius in the 1856 divorce case filed by Jonathan Miesse against Anna (a case later withdrawn).

24. Leavitt, "'A Worrying Profession'"; Barlow and Powell, "To Find a Stand." Nearly all small-town and rural physicians sought income elsewhere—as farmers, preachers, educators, or craftsmen—because of the economic vulnerability of their profession. In the nearby Maumee Valley, for example, local physicians also worked in real estate, banking, farming, and lumbering, and one operated a tavern. Wendler, "Doctors and Diseases," 228.

25. "In those days the doctor's office was generally attached to the residence, and the doctor's wife had to perform the duties of clerk as well as hostess to the various patrons seeking attention and relief" (*Indiana County*, 785).

26. Seidensticker, *The History of Medicine*, 8.

27. Ireland, *A History*, 8.

28. Jones, *An Historical Geography*, 23–24.

29. Schultz, "Divorce in Early America." Starting in 1843, local Ohio courts had the power to grant divorce, which meant that Jonathan could file for divorce in his local court rather than appeal to the entire assemblage of the Ohio State Legislature in Columbus—and he took advantage of this geographical and undoubtedly social and economic convenience in both 1849 and 1856.

30. *Miesse v. Miesse*, Common Plea Court, February 5, 1856, Wisconsin Historical Society.

31. Ibid.

32. Hartog, *Man and Wife*, 77.

33. Silkenat, *Moments of Despair*, 81.

34. Little, "A Woman of Property"; Shammas, "Re-assessing." The 1850 census had estimated the value of Jonathan's real estate at $12,000. Subtracting debts and other obligations, $3,000 may have been a rough equivalent of the one-third dower right (the part of an estate designated to provide support to a widow after her husband's death).

35. Hartog, *Man and Wife*, 76–87.

36. One of the few other reasons husbands gave wives property in their own name was to protect money from debts accrued by the husband. There is no evidence of this in this case.

37. *Miesse v. Miesse*, 1856.

38. Miesse, *A Journey*, preface and p. 3; *Miesse v. Miesse*, 1856. Jonathan departed Marseilles in March 1855 and had returned to Paris by June.

39. Passport application of Anna Miesse, Passport Applications, 1795–1905, at Fold3, accessed www.fold3.com/image/52200433?xid=1945, February 6, 2017 (hereafter known as Anna Miesse passport application).

40. Dickens, *Bleak House*, 624.

Chapter 2. The Questions of 1855

1. *Miesse v. Miesse*, 1856.

2. Ibid.; school student listings, Ohio Wesleyan University, 1854–55, U.S., School Catalogs, 1765–1935, Ancestry.com, 2012, accessed February 16, 2017.

3. Jonathan alleged, however, that upon his departure from town Anna took Aurelia "away from school" (*Miesse v. Miesse*, 1856).

4. Anna Miesse passport application.

5. Ibid.

6. Ibid.

7. Rosa Leinuel Kemball, Ohio, http://brianaltonenmph.com/6-history-of-medicine-and-pharmacy/eclectic-medicine-eclectics-1845–1875/, accessed February 5, 2017.

8. Robertson, *The Passport in America*, 168, 150.

Chapter 3. Miesse v. Miesse, *1856*

1. Hartog, *Man and Wife*, 66.

2. Schultz, "Divorce in Early America," 516–17.

3. *Miesse v. Miesse*, 1856. The specific timing of Anna's return to the United States and to Chillicothe is unclear, but on October 1 she purchased more land in Illinois.

4. Ibid.

5. While I've organized charges against Anna around four themes, the divorce complaint has no such organization.

6. *Miesse v. Miesse*, 1856.

7. For example: "On another occasion in the month of December last, in complainant's house, without provocation, violently attacked complainant, and beat him with a broom handle severely wounding one of his hands; On another occasion in January last, in complainant's house she attacked him with violent abuse, and threw a heavy knife at his head with great force, which if he had not sprung aside, would have inflicted a dangerous wound in his face; On several other occasions since her return she has attacked complainant, in his office, with a fire poker and other weapons, threatening to kill him, but was prevented by complainant and others" (ibid.).

8. Ibid.

9. Ibid.

10. Ibid., emphasis added.

11. Buckley, *The Great Catastrophe*, 195.

12. *Miesse v. Miesse*, 1856.

13. Ibid.

14. With the help of economist Vaskar Pahari, this financial equivalency is developed from Reinhart and Rogoff, *This Time Is Different.*

15. Basch, *Framing American Divorce*, 134; Grossberg, "Who Gets the Child?"; Hartog, "Lawyering." A close look at one divorce case is Grossberg, *A Judgement for Solomon.*

16. *Miesse v. Miesse*, 1856. The court required Anna to support Aurelia when Aurelia lived with her and required that Anna not take the child out of the country.

17. Hartog, *Man and Wife*, 139.

18. Ibid., 22, 75; Basch, *Framing American Divorce*, 103.

19. Silkenat, *Moments of Despair*, 80.

20. *Miesse v. Miesse*, 1856.

21. Ibid.

22. Silkenat, *Moments of Despair*, 81, 83.

23. *Miesse v. Miesse*, 1856.

24. Buckley, *The Great Catastrophe*, 200.

25. Silkenat, *Moments of Despair*, 85–86.

26. Ibid., 86.

Chapter 4. The Questions of 1856

1. George F. S. Ott is sometimes referred to as George T. S. Ott. Despite my best efforts I've been unable to find a birth date or location for George F. S. Ott or a death date or location for Sophia.

2. One record indicates May 11, 1856, as the marriage date. Another indicates June 1, 1856, as the marriage date.

3. Minetta Minona's name suggests a familiarity with Madison, Wisconsin. Madison is situated around and between two lakes: Lake Mendota and Lake Monona. When Anna and George built a stately mansion in 1859 they did so right on the shore of Lake Monona, and it was in that home that Minetta grew up. The name Minetta Minona is remarkably similar to Mendota and Monona. The meaning of the naming of Minetta Minona only suggests that someone saddled a young girl with a name that many in her community might consider ridiculous.

Chapter 5. Dr. Anna B. Ott, Local Doctress

1. Haltunnen, *Confidence Men*, 35.

2. Dane County, Wisconsin, population: 1846, 626; 1850, 1,672; 1855, 8,664; 1860, 6,611; 1865, 9,191; 1870, 9,176; 1875, 10,093; 1880, 10,841 (*A History of Dane County*, 728, 760).

3. Ibid., 609, 727, 763, 464.

4. Griswold, *Family and Divorce*, 19.

5. Del Mar, *What Trouble*, 5; Basch, *Framing American Divorce.*

6. Sager, *Marital Cruelty*, 55.

7. *A History of Dane County*, 1079. George V. Ott should not be confused with John

George Ott, a builder and the owner of a grocery store and brick business. Both men arrived in Madison at approximately the same time.

8. An image of the house from 1920 is available at http://www.wisconsinhistory.org/Content.aspx?dsNav=N:4294963828-4294955414&dsRecordDetails=R:IM43963. East Wilson Street is between Pinckney and Wisconsin Avenues; the Madison Terrace Hilton now sits at this address. Sometimes the address is listed as 96 East Wilson.

9. Alice and Bettina Jackson, "Architectural Styles in Pioneering Madison," folder 26, "Madison architecture," box 5, MSS 919, Jackson-Stevens-Morris Family Manuscript Collection, Wisconsin Historical Society, Madison. Compiled as a 1917 thesis and later published in the *Wisconsin State Journal*, May 6, 1923.

10. According to the 1860 census. Minetta is not mentioned in the 1860 census.

11. In 1857 eighteen physicians are recorded in Madison, divided as allopathic, homeopathic, and eclectic. *A History of Dane County*, 731.

12. Anna B. Ott v. George V. Ott, Dane County Circuit Court (Wisconsin), 1870 (hereafter cited as *Ott v. Ott*, 1870).

13. Thayer, "First in Their Class," 51–52. She was later married to Erastus B. Wolcott, Wisconsin's surgeon general during the Civil War. The Medical Society of Milwaukee organized in 1846. Harstad, "Frontier Medicine," 20–21.

14. In the Matter of the Motion to admit Miss Lavinia Goodell to the Bar of this Court, 39 Wis. 232 (1875), 244–45.

15. For a strong analysis of the reception of *Sex in Education*, see Hamlin, *From Eve to Evolution*, 73–733.

16. Clarke, *Sex in Education*, 105.

17. Fisher, *Plain Talk*, 24, 33.

18. *A History of Dane County*, 760 (see also 245).

19. Risse, "From Horse and Buggy," 29. See also Coombs, "Rural Medical Practice."

20. I'm concluding this based on the accusation that she robbed the Wells Fargo office after delivering a baby on September 8, 1857.

21. Receipt from Dunning and Sumner, Druggists, October 25, 1872, folders 2 and 3, box 1022, WIHV89-A940 Dane Series 121, Guardianship and Insanity Files, 1846–1925, Wisconsin County Court (Dane County) (hereafter cited as Guardianship Files).

22. Basch, *Framing American Divorce*, 102. Historian Norma Basch's research on New York in this period shows that over 60 percent of successful divorces were initiated by women.

23. Anna B. Ott v. George V. Ott, 1859 G., State of Wisconsin Circuit Court for Dane County, Wisconsin Historical Society (hereafter cited as *Ott v. Ott*, 1859).

24. Buckley, *The Great Catastrophe*, 192.

25. *Ott v. Ott*, 1859.

26. Buckley, *The Great Catastrophe*, 180.

27. Sager, *Marital Cruelty*, 129.

28. *Ott v. Ott*, 1859.

29. Ibid.

30. Ibid.

31. *Cincinnati Gazette*, January 28, 1868. See also *Cincinnati Gazette*, September 28, 1867.

32. The 1870 census lists two sons for Mrs. D. A. Smith: Charles, fourteen, and William, nine.

33. The *Daily Milwaukee News*, *Madison Journal*, *Janesville Gazette*, June 16, 1868; *Nashville Union and Dispatch*, June 18, 1868; *Sacramento Union*, July 7, 1868; *Madison Journal*, June 11, 1868; *Cincinnati Enquirer*, June 18, 1868; *Daily Milwaukee News*, June 13, 1868.

34. *Ott v. Ott*, 1870.

35. Buckley, *The Great Catastrophe*, 192.

36. *Ott v. Ott*, 1870.

37. Historian Robin Sager suggests that the frontier culture of Wisconsin resulted in violence of a more fierce nature than that in either Texas or Virginia: "All in all, the actions of cruel husbands and wives in Wisconsin led to more permanent injuries and generalized brutality within marriages than can be seen in either Virginia or Texas for the period" (*Marital Cruelty*, 39). See also Ramsey, "Domestic Violence"; and Ramsey, "The Exit Myth."

38. Fuentes, *Dispossessed Lives*, 146–47.

39. *Ott v. Ott*, 1870.

40. Siegel, "'The Rule of Love,'" 2130.

41. *Ott v. Ott*, 1870.

42. Ibid.

43. Ibid.

44. Ibid.

45. Ibid.

46. Ibid.

47. Harris, *State of the Marital Union*, 13–14.

48. *Ott v. Ott*, 1870.

49. Ibid.

50. Ibid.

51. Ibid. Stein worked in the house from October 1868 through at least January 1869 and is the focus of two depositions. Both were taken on December 24, 1868, the day after Anna filed for divorce. Though Stein did not understand the words when George spoke German, "his manner of tone and action showed plainly that he was angry."

52. *Ott v. Ott*, 1870.

53. *Wisconsin State Journal*, April 18, 1870, April 20, 1870, April 22, 1870, April 26, 1870, April 28, 1870.

54. Between 1874 and 1880 Aurelia divorced her husband, Dayton Morgan.

55. Josephine Waldschaky v. Anna B. Ott and George V. Ott, Wisconsin Circuit Court, 1871.

56. For more on the AMSAII, see Mohr, *Doctors and the Law*; Tomes, "The Great Restraint Controversy."

57. "Proceedings," 139, 166, 223, 260.

58. Ibid., 241, 258.

59. Ibid., 187, 191, 192, 242.

60. Mohr, *Doctors and the Law*, 164, and chap. 12.

61. Tomes, "The Great Restraint Controversy," 291; Mohr, *Doctors and the Law*, 167. Examples of exposés include Isaac Hunt, *Three Years in a Mad House* (1852); Francis Delilez, *The True Cause of Insanity Explained; or, The Terrible Experiences of an Insane, Related by Himself: The Life of a Patient in an Insane Asylum* (1888); Henry T. Helmbold, *Am I a Lunatic?* (1877); William L. Trully, *An Inner View of the State Lunatic Asylum at Utica* (1881); John A. Joyce, *A Checkered Life* (1883); Elizabeth Packard's writings; Anna Agnew, *From under the Cloud; or, Personal Reminiscences of Insanity* (1887); Clarissa C. Lathrop, *A Secret Institution* (1890); Rose and Barbara Trautman, *Wisconsin's Shame* (1892).

62. Carlisle, *Elizabeth Packard*, 158. For more on Packard, see Mohr, *Doctors and the Law*, 165–69.

63. Geller and Harris, *Women of the Asylum*, 61.

64. Quoted in ibid., xvii.

65. Packard, *Marital Power*, 7.

66. Ranney had been superintendent at Mendota, lost his position, and accepted another in Iowa.

67. "Proceedings," 249–250. Iowa law also required that all patients be given the names and addresses of the board members, and hospital personnel had no right to read or intervene in patients' mail.

68. Ibid., 250, 251.

69. Ibid., 258, 259.

70. *Wisconsin State Journal*, February 27, 1869; *Madison Daily Democrat*, February 27, 1869; Youmans, "How Wisconsin Women."

71. Hull, *The Woman Who Dared.*

72. Custer, "The Suffrage Battle."

73. Hull, *The Woman Who Dared*, 65.

74. *Wisconsin State Journal*, November 8, 1872.

75. Hull, *The Woman Who Dared.*

76. Cleary, "Married Women's Property Rights." Married women did not have the right to own property until 1850 or to control their earnings until 1872.

Chapter 6. Anna Ott, Insane Asylum Inmate

1. Series 2194, Mendota Mental Health Institute, Admissions, 1860–1908, box 4, admission no. 1763, Anna B. Ott, admitted May 12, 1873, Wisconsin Historical Society (hereafter cited as Series 2194).

2. *Reports of the Trustees*, 13.

3. *Annual Report 1860*, 24, 3.

4. Tomes, *A Generous Confidence*; Dwyer, *Homes for the Mad*. AMSAII is the precursor to the American Psychiatric Association.

5. Tomes, *A Generous Confidence,* 265.

6. *Reports of the Trustees,* 7. For more on the building and architecture of institutions, see Campbell, "Building Sanity"; Reiss, *Theaters of Madness*; Miron, *Prisons, Asylums, and the Public.*

7. Doherty, *The Best Specimen*; Brian, "'The Weight.'"

8. *Appendix to Annual Report,* 15, 17, 26, 41.

9. Ibid., 125–26.

10. Series 2194.

11. *Ott v. Ott,* 1870.

12. Carlisle, *Elizabeth Packard,* 7.

13. Packard, *Marital Power Exemplified,* 7.

14. Carlisle, *Elizabeth Packard,* 60.

15. Tomes, *A Generous Confidence,* 118, 121.

16. Grob, *Mental Illness,* 9.

17. *Annual Report 1861,* 1–2.

18. "Proceedings," 250, 251.

19. Tomes, *A Generous Confidence,* 118–28; Fox, *So Far Disordered,* 37–74.

20. Series 2171, Mendota Mental Health Institute, Patient Records, male/female 1860–1908, vol. 3, pp. 46–48, 498, admission no. 1763, Anna B. Ott, admitted May 12, 1873, Wisconsin Historical Society (hereafter cited as Series 2171).

21. Ibid. That this is in the medical records and not at all indicated in the legal records is interesting.

22. Nielsen, "Property, Disability."

23. Guardianship Files.

24. August 7, 1893, Series 2171. Also noted was that "among her delusions here is that of imagining her trunk being broken open, her clothing taken, worn and returned dirty, etc."

25. Guardianship Files.

26. August 14, 1873, Series 2171.

27. Usually listed as September 5, 1873, but occasionally listed as September 3, 1837.

28. "William W. Tredway." In the 1870s the Dane County court turned to him to serve as guardian to several others lacking appropriate family to do so. All the others were minor children.

29. Series 2171.

30. Series 2168, Mendota Mental Health Institute, Statistical Register, 1860–94, RLIN WIHV88-A409, Wisconsin Historical Society (hereafter cited as Series 2168).

31. Jimenez, *Changing Faces,* 69.

32. Tomes, *A Generous Confidence,* 195–96.

33. Rush, *Medical Inquiries,* 59–60.

34. Fisher, *Plain Talk,* 33.

35. Hamilton, *Types of Insanity,* introduction, 1, 3, plate V. See also Dwyer, *Homes for the Mad,* 5.

36. *Annual Report 1877,* 34.

37. Grob, *Mental Illness*, 8.

38. This later became Winnebago State Hospital and is now the Winnebago Mental Health Institute.

39. Series 2168.

40. For more on the link between civic fitness and mental fitness, see Waggoner, "'Oh Say Can You'"; Nielsen, "Helen Keller"; Minich, *Accessible Citizenships*.

41. Eli Clare has profoundly affected my thinking on diagnosis. As he has eloquently argued, "It is impossible to name all the ways in which diagnosis is useful. It propels eradication and affirms what we know about our own bodyminds. It extends the reach of genocide and makes meaning of the pain that keeps us up night after night. It allows for violence in the name of care and creates access to medical technology, human services, and essential care. It sets in motion social control and guides treatment that provides comfort. It takes away self-determination and saves lives. It disregards what we know about our own body-minds and leads to cure" (*Brilliant Imperfection*, 48).

42. Series 2168.

43. *First Biennial Report*, 9.

44. *Annual Report 1875*, 16.

45. "Mendota Chronicle: A Short History of Mendota State Hospital, 1960," manuscript written by the Centennial Committee at the Wisconsin Historical Society.

46. Dwyer, *Homes for the Mad*, 76.

47. Ray, *Ideal Characters*, 18.

48. *Rules and Regulations*, 7.

49. Dwyer, *Homes for the Mad*, 164.

50. Tomes, *A Generous Confidence*, 271.

51. Dwyer, *Homes for the Mad*, 17, 164. See also Grob, *Mental Illness*, 20; Grob, *The Mad among Us*, 95; Tomes, *A Generous Confidence*, 179–87. Chapter 3 in Reaume, *Remembrance of Patients Past*, paints a rich picture of daily institutional life in the Toronto Hospital for the Insane.

52. *Rules and Regulations*, 3–4.

53. *Annual Report 1873*, 41–42.

54. *Appendix*, 26, 73, 68, 75.

55. Tomes, *A Generous Confidence*, 273–74.

56. Series 2171.

57. March 6, 1874, Series 2171.

58. Ibid.

59. November 11, 1876, Series 2171. For more on violence in asylums, see Dwyer, *Homes for the Mad*, chap. 1.

60. December 16, 1873, November 11, 1876, October 29, 1880, March 30, 1881, Series 2171.

61. August 4, 1874, Series 2171. See also August 24, 1874, Series 2171: "A little imperious of late, assisting on the hall in her way, such as combing patients hair etc., etc."

62. Series 2171.

63. George V. Ott v. Anna B. Ott, State of Wisconsin, County of Dane, 1881, Wisconsin Historical Society (hereafter cited as *Ott v. Ott*, 1881).

64. October 29, 1880, Series 2171.

65. August 6, 1873, Series 2171.

66. January 6, 1874, Series 2171.

67. January 6, 1874, Series 2171.

68. On November 16, 1873, George Ott told Superintendent Ramsey that he would be visiting Mendota. See Series 1367, Mendota State Hospital, General Correspondence, box 11, February 1875–July 1875, Mental Hygiene (hereafter cited as Series 1367 plus the box and date range).

69. *Appendix to Annual Report*; *Report of the Committee.*

70. Burch, "Disorderly Pasts," 371.

71. *First Biennial Report*, 7.

72. Series 2171.

73. October 20, 1873, Series 2171.

74. June 20, 1874, Series 2171.

75. April 1, 1882, Series 2171.

76. November 5, 1883, Series 2171.

77. *First Biennial Report*, 6–7.

78. Thomas O'Kelly to Superintendent McDill, July 10, 1873, Series 1367, box 11, February 1875–July 1875.

79. March 5, 1875 from Angelina York to Superintendent Ranney, Series 1367.

80. Trautman and Trautman, *Wisconsin's Shame*, 11, 45, 46.

81. August 4, 1875, Series 2171.

82. December 1, 1875, and December 7, 1875, Series 2171.

83. Redjinski, "The Utica Crib"; Joinson, "The Perception and Treatment"; Bazar, "The Utica Crib."

84. Tomes, "The Great Restraint Controversy." For a discussion of restraint debates at the Toronto Hospital for the Insane, see Reaume, *Remembrance of Patients Past*, 14–15.

85. December 30, 1875, Series 2171.

86. *American Journal of Insanity* 31 (1874): 164.

87. Hubert, *Questions of Power*, 46.

88. *Report of the Committee*, 4.

89. Ibid., 59.

90. *Second Biennial Report*, 67–68.

91. *Fourth Annual Biennial Report.*

92. Geller and Harris, *Women of the Asylum*, 80.

93. Ibid., 51, 71, 56. Tirzah F. Shedd had similar warnings about her in her 1865 publication (ibid., 83).

94. Trautman and Trautman, *Wisconsin's Shame*, 15, 18.

95. Geller and Harris, *Women of the Asylum*, 54.

96. Ibid., 51.

97. Bly, *Ten Days in a Madhouse*, 88.

98. Geller and Harris, *Women of the Asylum*, 6.

99. "In most cases, Kirkbride could effectively counter the patient's claims by simply reminding patrons that the dissatisfied parties were in fact insane and characterizing their complaints as delusions" (Tomes, *A Generous Confidence*, 250).

100. *Annual Report 1875*, 15; *Second Biennial Report*, 76. In 1877 Superintendent Boughton blamed the killing of one patient by another on the hospital being "extremely crowded" (*Annual Report 1877*, 16, 17).

101. August 4, 1875, December 1, 7, 1875.

102. Geller and Harris, *Women of the Asylum*, 74.

103. Beaudreau and Finger, "Medical Electricity."

104. For more information on historians and HIPPA, see Lawrence, "Access Anxiety." According to the Wisconsin Historical Society website, "The State Archives does not meet the definition of a covered entity as defined by Health and Human Services (HHS) under the Health Insurance Portability and Accountability Act of 1996 (HIPAA). Access to health records at the WHS is governed by Wis. Stats. 146.85" (https://www.wisconsinhistory.org/Records/Article/CS15450, accessed March 5, 2018); Noll, "Patient Records."

105. Samuels, "Examining Millie and Christine McKoy." See also Burch, "'Dislocated Histories'"; Richards and Burch, "Documents."

106. *Annual Report 1874*, 5.

107. Series 2171.

108. March 30, 1881, Series 2171.

109. Stamp, "Wisconsin's Marriage and Divorce Laws," 103.

110. *Ott v. Ott*, 1881. The third physician was Dr. Clark Gapin.

111. Lunbeck, *The Psychiatric Persuasion*, 102–7.

112. *Ott v. Ott*, 1881.

113. Within a year the legislature overturned the law, making insanity no longer a legitimate grounds for divorce. See Schneider, "Unsoundness of Mind." George left Madison in 1883 for Florida. I have been unable to trace him there. See *Wisconsin State Journal*, November 14, 1923.

114. *Annual Report 1876*, 21.

115. March 30, 1881, receipt. Anna B. Ott Guardianship and Insanity Files, Dane Series 121.

Chapter 7. Anna Ott, Economic Agent

1. *Annual Report 1873*. This included five officers, one gardener, sixteen male attendants, eighteen female attendants, five laborers, one launderer, eight laundresses, one butcher, one baker, one male and one female night watchman, one coachman, seven cooks and assistants, two seamstresses, two carpenters, one male and one female supervisor, two chambermaids, one chaplain, one porter, one engineer, one engineer's assistant, one painter, one fireman, one farmer, and two waiters.

2. This financial equivalency is developed from Reinhart and Rogoff, *This Time Is Different*, with the help of economist Vaskar Pahari.

3. October 14, 1875, receipt from John N. Jones, Wagon and Carriage Stock, work on roof, $9.00; April 30, 1877, receipt for cleaning privy vault at store, $2.50; January 30, 1880, receipt for sidewalk repairs, $6.30; all in Guardianship Files.

4. December 1, 1874, Guardianship Files.

5. Statement of receipts from March 31, 1877 through March 1, 1879 (twenty-three months), November 9, 1881, Guardianship Files.

6. March 28, 1883, Guardianship Files.

7. April 30, 1878, July 16, 1879, December 20, 1880, Guardianship Files.

8. Guardianship Files.

9. For clothing expenses, see April 11, 1874, November 21, 1875, March 20, 1876, April 7, 1876, June 10, 1876, October 14, 1876, December 4, 1876, March 1877, March 29, 1877, April 25, 1877, July 20, 1877, August 3, 1877, August 6, 1877, December 20, 1877, February 7, 1878, February 25, 1878, April 25, 1878, May 20, 1878, September 16, 1878, October 17, 1878, November 19, 1878, December 7, 1878, January 18, 1879, July 26, 1879, Oct 1, 1879, December 26, 1879, January 10, 1880, March 31, 1880, July 21, 1880, July 31, 1880, February 4, 1881, April 5, 1881, June 10, 1881, June 17, 1881, July 23, 1881, Guardianship Files. For food expenses, see January 6, 1874, July 30, 1874, March 26, 1877, April 22, 1878, March 1879, March 29, 1880, January 17, 1881, December 21, 1881, Guardianship Files.

10. April 11, 1874, Guardianship Files.

11. December 4, 1876, Guardianship Files.

12. Receipt, February 4, 1881, Guardianship Files.

13. March 29, 1880, George W. Huntley, Grocer, Guardianship Files.

14. January 29, 1883, J. H. D. Baker, Groceries, Crockery and Seeds, Guardianship Files.

15. Lizzie Hess to Dr. McDill, May 31, 1875, Series 1367.

16. Case of Reuben Fairman, Dane County Guardianship and Insanity Files, DCPCC box 1028 (box 4, folder 5).

17. For a discussion of the relationship between labor and disability definitions, see Nielsen, "Incompetent and Insane."

18. *Annual Report 1876*, 17.

19. Ibid., 17.

20. *First Biennial Report*, 8.

21. January 15, 1884, Series 2171.

22. *Report of the Committee*, 19.

23. *Ott v. Ott*, 1881.

24. *Annual Report 1874*, 23.

25. George Ott to Dr. Ranney, November 16, 1873 (box 8); D. Morgan to Superintendent, October 30, 1874 (box 10); A. Morgan to Mr. Tredway, July 30, 1876, all in Series 1367.

26. Note, September 10, 1879; A. Morgan to Tredway, September 13, 1879; A. Morgan to Tredway, September 26, 1879, all in Guardianship Files.

27. Series 1367.

28. Mrs. Cyrene Green to Dear Sir, May 12, 1874, Series 1367.

29. D. A. Davis to Dr. McDill, May 11, 1875, Series 1367.

30. Charles Dobb to Dr. McDill, October 8, 1872; John Bentley to Mark Ranney, April 4, 1874, both in Series 1367.

31. Marie Allen to Dr. McDill, October 21, 1872, box 6, October 1872–May 1873; Louis Blank to Dr. Mark Ranney, April 4, 1874, box 9, April 1874–August 1874; Edward Bishop to Mark Ranney, May 7, 1874, all in Series 1367.

32. Edgar Ray to Dear Sir, May 6, 1876, Series 1367.

33. Elisa Bright to Dr. McDill, October 17, 1873, Series 1367.

34. Dora Servis to Mr. McDill, May 23, 1875, Series 1367.

35. S. S. Luscombe to Dr. Mark Ranney, November 3, 1873, Series 1367.

36. For example, Lizzie Hess to Dr. McDill, May 31, 1875; Henry Mathans to Dear Sir, March 29, 1875, both in Series 1367.

37. Miss L. M. Williams, February 18, 1876, Series 1367.

38. Emily Sandford, April 25, 1874, Series 1367.

39. Miletus Knight, October 20, 1875, Series 1367.

40. For example, Mrs. Charles Finch, May 15, 1874, Series 1367.

41. B. W. Doyle to Dr. Ranney, Series 1367.

42. Peter Kavenaugh to Dr. Ranney, April 12, 1874, Series 1367.

43. Andrews, "President's Address," 51.

Chapter 8. Remembering Anna Ott

1. *Sixth Biennial Report*, 55. In general, hospital personnel across the nation struggled to rid institutions of infectious and potentially deadly diseases such as cholera, dysentery, and flu. Violence happened, accidents happened, and people grew older.

2. August Wilde to Mark Ranney, Milwaukee, June 22, 1874, Series 1367, General Correspondence, Mendota State Hospital, box 9, April 1874–August 1874. According to the 1880 census, a Henrietta Pahl resided in the Milwaukee Insane Asylum.

3. J. W. Bates, Office of Bates & Nichols, Attorneys at Law, to Supt Insane Asylum, November 18, 1876, box 13, May 1876–December 1876, Series 1367.

4. For a sampling, see "A Deathbed Confession," *Alexandria (VA) Gazette*, September 4, 1893, 1; "Confessed on Her Deathbed," *Cedar Rapids (IA) Evening Gazette*, August 31, 1893, 1; "A Dying Confession," *Cincinnati Enquirer*, August 31, 1893, 5; "Woman Robbed the Express Company," *Columbus (IN) Daily Herald*, August 31, 1893, 1; "She Confessed the Robbery," *St. Paul Daily Globe*, September 2, 1893, 6; "A Dying Confession," *Xenia (OH) Daily Gazette*, September 1, 1893, 1.

5. See the description of the Ott-Wright house at http://www.wisconsinhistory.org/Content.aspx?dsNav=Ny:True,N:4294963828-4294955414&dsNavOnly=N:1135&dsRecordDetails=R:IM43963, accessed March 8, 2016. See also Alice and Bettina Jackson, "Architectural Styles in Pioneering Madison," unpublished manuscript compiled

as a 1917 thesis in a postgraduate course in house planning at UW under Miss Abby Marlatt, head of the Home Economics Department. Published in the *Wisconsin State Journal*, May 6, 1923, MS 919, folder 26, box 5, Madison Architecture, Jackson-Stevens-Morris Family Manuscript Collection, Wisconsin Historical Society.

6. Baynton, "Disability"; Pitts, "Disability"; Cogan, "The Look Within."

7. Rosenberg, "The Tyranny of Diagnosis," 243. For other analyses of diagnosis, see Hacking, "Kinds of People"; Arnaud, *On Hysteria*, esp. chap. 2.

8. Chamberlain, *The Notorious Elizabeth Tuttle.*

9. Lunbeck, *The Psychiatric Persuasion,* 147.

10. For an example of an insanity diagnosis used to gain property, see Andrews, *Insane Sisters.*

11. Cahn, "Border Disorders," 260.

12. Nasaw, "Introduction," 573; Banner, "AHR Roundtable," 580.

13. Nielsen, "The Perils." Ann M. Little makes a strong case for biography in *The Many Captivities*, 9–15.

14. Price, "The Bodymind Problem"; Donaldson, "Revisiting"; Cahn, "Border Disorders," 260, 275; Mollow, "Mad Feminism"; Rodas, "PreOccupied."

15. Chesler, *Women and Madness*; Gilbert and Gubar, *The Madwoman in the Attic.*

Bibliography

Abrahams, Harold J. *Extinct Medical Schools of Nineteenth-Century Philadelphia.* Philadelphia: University of Pennsylvania Press, 1966.

Andrews, Gregg. *Insane Sisters: Or, the Price Paid for Challenging a Company Town.* Columbia: University of Missouri Press, 1999.

Andrews, J. B. "President's Address before the American Medico-Psychological Association." *American Journal of Insanity* 50, no. 1 (July 1893): 49–60.

Annual Report of the Board of Trustees of the Wisconsin State Hospital for the Insane for the Year 1860. Madison: James Ross, State Printer, 1860.

Annual Report of the Board of Trustees of the Wisconsin State Hospital for the Insane for the Year 1861. Madison: James Ross, State Printer, 1861.

Annual Report of the Board of Trustees of the Wisconsin State Hospital for the Insane for the Year Ending September 30, 1873. Madison: James Ross, State Printer, 1873.

Annual Report of the Board of Trustees of the Wisconsin State Hospital for the Insane for the Year Ending September 30, 1974. Madison: James Ross, State Printer, 1874.

Annual Report of the Board of Trustees of the Wisconsin State Hospital for the Insane for the Year Ending September 30, 1875. Madison: James Ross, State Printer, 1875.

Annual Report of the Board of Trustees of the Wisconsin State Hospital for the Insane for the Year Ending September 30, 1876. Madison: James Ross, State Printer, 1876.

Annual Report of the Board of Trustees of the Wisconsin State Hospital for the Insane for the Year Ending September 30, 1877. Madison: James Ross, State Printer, 1877.

Appendix to Annual Report of the State Hospital for the Insane for the Year 1868. Madison: James Ross, State Printer, 1868.

Arnaud, Sabine. *On Hysteria: The Invention of a Medical Category between 1670 and 1820.* Chicago: University of Chicago Press, 2016.

Banner, Lois. "AHR Roundtable, Historians and Biography." *American Historical Review* 114, no. 3 (June 2009): 579–86.

Barlow, William, and David O. Powell. "To Find a Stand: New England Physicians on the Western and Southern Frontier." *Bulletin of the History of Medicine* 54, no. 3 (Fall 1980): 386–401.

Basch, Norma. *Framing American Divorce: From the Revolutionary Generation to the Victorians.* Berkeley: University of California Press, 1999.

Baynton, Douglas. 2001. "Disability and the Justification of Inequality in American History." In *The New Disability History: American Perspectives*, ed. Paul K. Longmore and Lauri Umansky, 33–57. New York: New York University Press.

Bazar, Jennifer L. "The Utica Crib: Biography of an Unknown Barbarous Object." *History of Psychology* 18, no. 2 (2015): 132–45.

Beaudreau, Sherry Ann, and Stanley Finger. "Medical Electricity and Madness in the 18th Century: The Legacies of Benjamin Franklin and Jan Ingenhousz." *Perspectives in Biology and Medicine* 49, no. 3 (Summer 2006): 330–45.

Beecher, Catharine. *A Treatise on Domestic Economy, for the Use of Young Ladies at Home, and at School.* New York: Harper and Brothers, 1846.

A Biographical History of Darke County, Ohio: Compendium of National Biography. Chicago: Lewis Publishing Company, 1900.

Bly, Nellie. *Ten Days in a Madhouse*. New York: Ian L. Munro, 1887.

Brian, Kathleen M. "'The Weight of Perhaps Ten or a Dozen Human Lives': Suicide, Accountability, and the Life-Saving Technologies of the Asylum." *Bulletin of the History of Medicine* 90, no. 4 (Winter 2016): 583–610.

Brown, Jeffrey P. "Chillicothe's Elite: Leadership in a Frontier Community." *Ohio History* 96 (Summer–Autumn 1987): 140–56.

Buckley, Thomas E. *The Great Catastrophe of My Life: Divorce in the Old Dominion.* Chapel Hill: University of North Carolina Press, 2002.

Burch, Susan. "'Dislocated Histories': The Canton Asylum for Insane Indians." *Women, Gender, and Families of Color* 2, no. 2 (Fall 2014): 141–62.

———. "Disorderly Pasts: Kinship, Diagnoses, and Remembering in American Indian-U.S. Histories." *Journal of Social History* 50, no. 2 (Winter 2016): 362–385.

Burch, Susan, and Hannah Joyner. *Unspeakable: The Story of Junius Wilson.* Chapel Hill: University of North Carolina Press, 2007.

Burman, Sondra. "Battered Women: Stages of Change and Other Treatment Models That Instigate and Sustain Leaving." *Treatment & Crisis Intervention* 3, no. 1 (Spring 2003): 83–98.

Cahn, Susan K. "Border Disorders: Mental Illness, Feminist Metaphor, and the Disordered Female Psyche in the Twentieth-Century United States." In *Disability Histories*, ed. Susan Burch and Michael Rembis, 258–81. Urbana: University of Illinois Press, 2014.

Campbell, Kim. "Building Sanity: The Rise and Fall of Architectural Treatment at the South Carolina Lunatic Asylum." *South Carolina Historical Magazine* 116, no. 2 (April 2015): 100–121.

Carlisle, Linda V. *Elizabeth Packard: A Noble Fight.* Urbana: University of Illinois Press, 2010.

Carter, Angela, "Teaching with Trauma: Trigger Warnings, Feminism, and Disability Pedagogy." *Disability Studies Quarterly* 35, no. 2 (2015).

Chamberlain, Ava. *The Notorious Elizabeth Tuttle: Marriage, Murder, and Madness in the Family of Jonathan Edwards*. New York: New York University Press, 2012.

Chesler, Phyllis. *Women and Madness.* Garden City, NJ: Doubleday, 1972.

Clare, Eli. *Brilliant Imperfection: Grappling with Cure.* Durham, NC: Duke University Press, 2017.

Clarke, Edward H. *Sex in Education, or, A Fair Chance for the Girls.* Boston: J. Osgood and Company, 1873.

Cleary, Catherine B. "Married Women's Property Rights in Wisconsin, 1846–1872." *Wisconsin Magazine of History* 78, no. 2 (1994–95): 110–37.

Cogan, Jacob Katz. 1997. "The Look Within: Property, Capacity, and Suffrage in Nineteenth-Century America." *Yale Law Journal* 107 (1997): 473–98.

Coombs, Jan. "Rural Medical Practice in the 1880s: A View from Central Wisconsin." *Bulletin of the History of Medicine* 64 (1990): 35–62.

Custer, Frank S. "The Suffrage Battle." *Madison Magazine,* September 1987, 93–96.

Del Mar, David Peterson. *What Trouble I Have Seen: A History of Violence against Wives.* Cambridge, MA: Harvard University Press, 1996.

Dickens, Charles. *Bleak House.* New York: Dover Thrift Edition, 2017.

Doherty, Thomas. *The Best Specimen of a Tyrant: The Ambitious Dr. Abraham Van Norstrand and the Wisconsin Insane Hospital.* Iowa City: University of Iowa Press, 2013.

Donaldson, Elizabeth J. "Revisiting the Corpus of the Madwoman: Further Notes toward a Feminist Disability Studies Theory of Mental Illness." In *Feminist Disability Studies*, ed. Kim Q. Hall, 91–113. Bloomington: Indiana University Press, 2011.

Dwyer, Ellen. *Homes for the Mad: Life inside Two Nineteenth-Century Asylums.* New Brunswick, NJ: Rutgers University Press, 1987.

Emerson, Jason. *The Madness of Mary Lincoln.* Carbondale: Southern Illinois University Press, 2007.

Epstein, Steven. *Inclusion: The Politics of Difference in Medical Research.* Chicago: University of Chicago Press, 2009.

First Biennial Report of the Wisconsin State Hospital for the Insane for the Two Fiscal Years Ending September 30, 1884. Madison: James Ross, State Printer, 1884.

Fisher, T. W. *Plain Talk about Insanity.* Boston: Alexander Moore, 1872.

Foucault, Michel. *Madness and Civilization: A History of Insanity in the Age of Reason.* New York: Vintage Books, 1988.

———. "Lives of Infamous Men." *Power Essential Works of Foucault, 1954–1984* (New York: The New Press, 2001), 162.

Fourth Annual Biennial Report of the State Board of Supervision of Wisconsin Charitable, Reformatory and Penal Institutions for the Two Fiscal Years Ending September 30, 1890. Madison: James Ross, State Printer, 1890.

Fox, Richard W. *So Far Disordered in Mind: Insanity in California, 1870–1930.* Berkeley: University of California Press, 1979.

Fuentes, Marisa J. *Dispossessed Lives: Enslaved Women, Violence, and the Archive.* Philadelphia: University of Pennsylvania Press, 2016.

Geller, Jeffrey L., and Maxine Harris. *Women of the Asylum: Voices from behind the Walls, 1840–1945.* New York: Anchor Books, 1994.

Gilbert, Sandra M., and Susan Gubar. *The Madwoman in the Attic: The Woman Writer and the Nineteenth-Century Literary Imagination.* New Haven, CT: Yale University Press, 1978.

Goffman, Erving. *Asylums: Essays on the Social Situation of Mental Patients and Other Inmates.* New York: Anchor Books, 1961.

Goodley, Dan. *Dis/Ability Studies: Theorising Disablism and Ableism.* London: Routledge Press, 2014.

Griswold, Robert L. 1982. *Family and Divorce in California, 1850–1890: Victorian Illusions and Everyday Realities.* Albany: State University of New York Press.

Grob, Gerald. *The Mad among Us: The History of the Care of America's Mentally Ill.* New York: Macmillan, 1984.

———. *Mental Illness and American Society, 1875–1940.* Princeton, NJ: Princeton University Press, 1983.

———. *Mental Institutions in America: Social Policy to 1875.* New York: Free Press, 1973.

Grossberg, Michael. *A Judgement for Solomon: The D'Haueteville Case and Legal Experiences in Antebellum America.* New York: Cambridge University Press, 1996.

———. "Who Gets the Child? Custody, Guardianship, and the Rise of a Judicial Patriarchy in Nineteenth-Century America." *Feminist Studies* 9 (1983): 235–60.

Hacking, Ian. "Kinds of People: Moving Targets." Tenth British Academy Lecture, April 11, 2006. https://www.britac.ac.uk/sites/default/files/hacking-draft.pdf.

Haltunnen, Karen. *Confidence Men and Painted Women: A Study of Middle-Class Culture in America, 1830–1870.* New Haven, CT: Yale University Press, 1982.

Hamilton, Allan McLane. *Types of Insanity: An Illustrated Guide to the Physical Diagnosis of Mental Disease.* New York: William Wood and Company, 1883.

Hamlin, Kimberly A. *From Eve to Evolution: Darwin, Science, and Women's Rights in Gilded Age America.* Chicago: University of Chicago Press, 2014.

Harris, Leslie J. *State of the Marital Union: Rhetoric, Identity, and Nineteenth-Century Marriage Controversies.* Waco, TX: Baylor University Press, 2014.

Harstad, Peter. "Frontier Medicine in the Territory of Wisconsin." In *Wisconsin Medicine: Historical Perspectives,* ed. Ronald L. Numbers and Judith Walzer Leavitt, 13–23. Madison: University of Wisconsin Press, 1981.

Hartman, Saidiya. "Venus in Two Acts." *small axe* 12, no. 2 (June 2008): 1–14.

Hartog, Hendrik. "Lawyering, Husbands' Rights, and 'the Unwritten Law' in Nineteenth-Century America." *Journal of American History* 84, no. 1 (June 1997): 67–96.

———. *Man and Wife in America: A History.* Cambridge, MA: Harvard University Press, 2000.

Heilbrun, Carolyn G. *Writing a Woman's Life.* New York: Ballantine, 1988.

A History of Dane County. Chicago: Western Historical Company, 1880.

History of Ross and Highland Counties, Ohio: Biographical Sketches. Cleveland: Williams Bros., Publishers, 1880.

Hixson, Walter L. *American Settler Colonialism: A History*. New York: Palgrave Macmillan, 2013.

Hubert, Susan J. *Questions of Power: The Politics of Women's Madness Narratives.* Newark: University of Delaware Press, 2002.

Hull, N. E. H. *The Woman Who Dared to Vote: The Trial of Susan B. Anthony.* Lawrence: University Press of Kansas, 2012.

Indiana County, Pennsylvania: Her People, Past and Present . . . Vol. 1. Chicago: J. H. Beers, 1913.

Ireland, A. C. *A History of the Chillicothe Fire Department, 1845–1880*. Chillicothe, OH: Ross County Historical Society Press, 1944.

Jimenez, Mary Ann. *Changing Faces of Madness: Early American Attitudes and Treatment of the Insane.* Lebanon, NH: University Press of New England, 1987.

Joinson, Carla. "The Perception and Treatment of Insanity in Southern Appalachia." MA thesis, East Tennessee State University, 2012.

Jones, Mary Somerville. *An Historical Geography of the Changing Divorce Law in the United States.* New York: Garland Publishing, Inc., 1987.

Kafer, Alison. *Feminist, Queer, Crip*. Bloomington: Indiana University Press, 2013.

Lawrence, Susan C. "Access Anxiety: HIPAA and Historical Research." *Journal of the History of Medicine and Allied Sciences* 62, no. 4 (2007): 422–60.

Leavitt, Judith Walzer. "'A Worrying Profession': The Domestic Environment of Medical Practice in Mid-Nineteenth-Century America." *Bulletin of the History of Medicine* 69, no. 1 (Spring 1995): 1–29.

Little, Ann M. *The Many Captivities of Esther Wheelright.* New Haven, CT: Yale University Press, 2016.

Little, Sarah Miller. "A Woman of Property: From Being It to Controlling It; A Bicentennial Perspective on Women and Ohio Property Law, 1803 to 2003." *Hasting Women's Law Journal* 16, no. 2 (Summer 2005): 177–200.

Lunbeck, Elizabeth. *The Psychiatric Persuasion: Knowledge, Gender, and Power in Modern America.* Princeton, NJ: Princeton University Press, 1994.

Metzl, Jonathan M. *The Protest Psychosis: How Schizophrenia Became a Black Disease.* Boston, MA: Beacon Press, 2009.

Metzl, Jonathan M., and Anna Kirkland, eds. *Against Health: How Health Became the New Morality.* New York: New York University Press, 2010.

Miesse, Jonathan. *A Journey to Egypt and Palestine, in the Year 1855.* Chillicothe, OH: Scioto Gazette, 1859.

Minich, Julie. *Accessible Citizenships: Disability, Nation, and the Cultural Politics of Greater Mexico.* Philadelphia: Temple University Press, 2013.

Miron, Jane. *Prisons, Asylums, and the Public: Institutional Visiting in the Nineteenth Century.* Toronto: University of Toronto Press, 2011.

Mohr, James C. *Doctors and the Law: Medical Jurisprudence in Nineteenth-Century America.* Baltimore, MD: Johns Hopkins University Press, 1993.

Mollow, Anna. "Mad Feminism." *Social Text*, October 24, 2013. Accessed June 1, 2018. https://socialtextjournal.org/periscope_article/mad-feminism/.

Nasaw, David. "Introduction: AHR Roundtable, Historians and Biography." *American Historical Review* 114, no. 3 (June 2009): 573–78.

Nielsen, Kim E. "Dr. Anna B. Ott, Patient #1763: The Messiness of Authority, Diagnosis, Gender, and Insanity in Nineteenth-Century America." *Signs* 45, no. 1 (Spring 2019): 27–49.

———. "Helen Keller and the Politics of Civic Fitness." In *The New Disability History: American Perspectives*, ed. Paul Longmore and Lauri Umansky, 268–90. New York: New York University Press, 2001.

———. "Incompetent and Insane: Labor, Ability, and Citizenship in Nineteenth- and Early-Twentieth-Century United States." *Rethinking History* 23, no. 2 (2019): 175–88.

———. "The Perils and Promises of Disability Biography." In *The Oxford Handbook of Disability History*, ed. Michael Rembis, Catherine Kudlick, and Kim E. Nielsen, 21–40. New York: Oxford University Press, 2018.

———. "Property, Disability, and the Making of the Incompetent Citizen in the United States, 1880s–1940s." In *Disability Histories*, ed. Susan Burch and Michael Rembis, 308–20. Urbana: University of Illinois Press, 2014.

Noll, Steven. "Patient Records and Historical Stories: The Case of Caswell Training School." *Bulletin of the History of Medicine* 68 (1994): 411–28.

Norwood, William Frederick. *Medical Education in the United States before the Civil War*. Philadelphia: University of Pennsylvania Press, 1944.

Packard, Elizabeth. *Marital Power Exemplified in Mrs. Packard's Trial and Self-Defense from the Charge of Insanity; or, Three Years Imprisonment for Religious Belief, by the Arbitrary Will of a Husband, with an Appeal to the Government to So Change the Laws as to Afford Legal Protection to Married Women*. Hartford, CT: Case, Lockwood, 1870.

Penney, Darby, and Peter Stastny. *The Lives They Left Behind: Suitcases from a State Hospital Attic*. New York: Bellevue Literary Press, 2009.

Pitts, Yvonne. "Disability, Scientific Authority, and Women's Political Participation in the Turn of the Twentieth Century United States." *Journal of Women's History* 22 (2012): 37–61.

Portrait and Biographical Record of the Scioto Valley, Ohio. Chicago: Lewis Publishing Company, 1894.

Price, Margaret. "The Bodymind Problem and the Possibilities of Pain." *Hypatia* 30, no. 1 (2015): 268–84.

"Proceedings of the Association of Medical Superintendents." *American Journal of Insanity*, October 1872, 137–263.

Ramsey, Carolyn B. "Domestic Violence and State Intervention in the American West and Australia, 1860–1930." *Indiana Law Journal* 86, no. 195 (2011): 185–255.

———. "The Exit Myth: Family Law, Gender Roles, and Changing Attitudes toward Female Victims of Domestic Violence." *Michigan Journal of Gender and Law* 200, no. 1 (2013): 1–32.

Ray, Isaac. *Ideal Characters of the Officers of a Hospital for the Insane, Read to the Association of Superintendents of North American Hospitals for the Insane, at Its Annual Meeting in Baltimore, May 29, 1873 and Ordered to Be Printed.* Philadelphia, 1873.

———. *Mental Hygiene.* Boston: Ticknor and Fields, 1863.

Reaume, Geoffrey. *Remembrance of Patients Past: Patient Life at the Toronto Hospital for the Insane, 1870–1940.* Toronto: Oxford University Press, 2000.

Redjinski, John. "The Utica Crib." *Bulletin of the Menninger Clinic* 35, no. 3 (May 1971): 202–6.

Reinhart, Carmen M., and Kenneth S. Rogoff. *This Time Is Different: Eight Centuries of Financial Folly.* Princeton, NJ: Princeton University Press, 2009.

Reiss, Benjamin. *Theaters of Madness: Insane Asylums and Nineteenth-Century American Culture.* Chicago: University of Chicago Press, 2008.

Report of the Committee Appointed under Provisions of Joint Resolution #33A, 1880, to Investigate into the Affairs of the Wisconsin State Hospital for the Insane. Madison: James Ross, State Printer, 1880.

Reports of the Trustees and Building Commissioners of the Wisconsin State Hospital for the Insane. Madison: James Ross, State Printer, 1859.

Reverby, Susan M. "Inclusion and Exclusion: The Politics of History, Difference, and Medical Research." *Journal of the History of Medicine and Allied Sciences* 63, no. 1 (January 2008): 103–13.

Richards, Penny L., and Susan Burch. "Documents, Ethics, and the Disability Historian." In *The Oxford Handbook of Disability History*, ed. Michael Rembis, Catherine Kudlick, and Kim E. Nielsen, 161–76. New York: Oxford University Press, 2018.

Rippley, Laverne J. "The Chillicothe Germans." *Ohio History* 74 (December 1966): 212–25.

Risse, Guenter B. "From Horse and Buggy to Automobile and Telephone: Medical Practice in Wisconsin, 1848–1930." In *Wisconsin Medicine: Historical Perspectives*, ed. Ronald L. Numbers and Judith Walzer Leavitt, 25–45. Madison: University of Wisconsin Press, 1981.

Robertson, Craig. *The Passport in America: The History of a Document.* New York: Oxford University Press, 2010.

Rodas, Julia Miele. "PreOccupied." *Social Text*, October 24, 2013. Accessed June 1, 2018. https://socialtextjournal.org/periscope_article/preoccupied/.

Rosenberg, Charles E. "The Tyranny of Diagnosis: Specific Entities and Individual Experience." *Milbank Quarterly* 80, no. 2 (2002): 237–60.

Rothman, David. *Conscience and Convenience: The Asylum and Its Alternatives in Progressive America.* Boston: Little, Brown, 1980.

———. *The Discovery of the Asylum: Social Order and Disorder in the New Republic.* Boston: Little, Brown and Company, 1971.

Rowe, Jill. "In Strength & Struggle: Free Black Communities in the Old Northwest." Paper presented at the conference "Africa and the Global Atlantic World," Kent State University, Kent, Ohio, 2016. Accessed June 29, 2018. https://www.researchgate

.net/publication/290997134_In_Strength_Struggle_Free_Black_Communities_in_the_Old_Northwest.

Rules and Regulations for the Government of Those Employed at the Wisconsin State Hospital for the Insane (1877). Hos M.1:1880, no. 3. Wisconsin Government Documents. Wisconsin Historical Society Library, Madison.

Rush, Benjamin. *Medical Inquiries and Observations upon the Diseases of the Mind.* 2nd ed. Philadelphia: Kimber and Richardson, 1818.

Sager, Robin C. *Marital Cruelty in Antebellum America.* Baton Rouge: Louisiana State University Press, 2016.

Salafia, Matthew. *Slavery's Borderland: Freedom and Bondage along the Ohio River.* Philadelphia: University of Pennsylvania Press, 2013.

Samuels, Ellen. "Examining Millie and Christine McKoy: Where Enslavement and Enfreakment Meet." *Signs* 37, no. 1 (2011): 53–81.

Schneider, John H. "Unsoundness of Mind as Ground for Divorce: A Proposal." *Wisconsin Law Review* 106 (May 1944): 109–10.

Schultz, Martin. "Divorce in Early America: Origins and Patterns in Three North Central States." *Sociological Quarterly* 25, no. 4 (Autumn 1984): 511–26.

Second Biennial Report of the State Board of Supervision of Wisconsin Charitable, Reformatory and Penal Institutions for the Two Fiscal Years Ending September 30, 1886. Madison: James Ross, State Printer, 1886.

Seidensticker, John. *The History of Medicine in Ross County, 1796–1994.* Chillicothe, OH: Medical Center Hospital, 1995.

Shammas, Carole. "Re-assessing the Married Women's Property Acts." *Journal of Women's History* 6, no. 1 (Spring 1994): 9–30.

Shryock, Richard Harrison. *Medical Licensing in America, 1650–1965.* Baltimore, MD: Johns Hopkins Press, 1967.

Siegel, Reva B. "'The Rule of Love': Wife Beating as Prerogative and Privacy." *Yale Law Journal* 105, no. 8 (June 1996): 2117–207.

Silkenat, David. *Moments of Despair: Suicide, Divorce, and Debt in Civil War Era North Carolina.* Chapel Hill: University of North Carolina Press, 2011.

Simplican, Stacy Clifford. "Feminist Disability Studies as Methodology: Life-Writing and the Abled/Disabled Binary." *Feminist Review* 3, no. 1 (2017): 46–60.

Sixth Biennial Report of the Wisconsin State Hospital for the Insane for the Two Fiscal Years Ending September 30, 1894. Madison: Democrat Printing Company, 1894.

Sklar, Kathryn Kish. *Catharine Beecher: A Study in American Domesticity.* New Haven, CT: Yale University Press, 1973.

Stamp, Mark A. "Wisconsin's Marriage and Divorce Laws: A Historical Perspective," ML Thesis, University of Wisconsin, 1982.

Szasz, Thomas. *The Myth of Mental Illness: Foundations of a Theory of Personal Conduct.* New York: Harper and Row, 1974.

Thayer, Earl R. "First in Their Class: Wisconsin's Pioneering Women Physicians." *Wisconsin Academy Review* 51, no. 2 (Spring 2005): 51–62.

Tomes, Nancy. *A Generous Confidence: Thomas Story Kirkbride and the Art of Asylum Keeping, 1840–1883*. New York: Cambridge University Press, 1984.

———. "The Great Restraint Controversy: A Comparative Perspective on Anglo-American Psychiatry in the Nineteenth-Century." In *Anatomy of Madness: Essays in the History of Psychiatry*, ed. W. F. Bynum, Roy Porter, and Michael Shepherd, 199–205. London: Routledge, 1985.

Trautman, Rose, and Barbara Trautman. *Wisconsin's Shame: Insane Asylums or the American Bastille! The Narrative of the Kidnapping of the Misses Trautman, of Sauk City, Wis., on a Sunday Afternoon, and Running Them into an Insane Asylum; Their Two Years' Shocking Experience and Observation in the State Hospitals at Mendota and Oshkosh*. Chicago: Guiding Star, 1892.

"William W. Tredway." In *The US Biographical Dictionary and Portrait Gallery of Eminent and Self-Made Men, Wisconsin Volume*. Chicago: American Biographical Publishing Company, 1877.

Waggoner, Jess. "'Oh Say Can You ___': Race and Mental Disability in Performances of Citizenship." *Journal of Literary and Cultural Disability Studies* 10, no. 1 (2016): 87–102.

Wendler, Marilyn Van Voorhis. "Doctors and Diseases on the Ohio Frontier." *Ohio History* 89, no. 2 (1980): 222–40.

Youmans, Theodora W. "How Wisconsin Women Won the Ballot." *Wisconsin Magazine of History* 5, no. 1 (September 1921): 3–32.

Index

KIM E. NIELSEN is a professor and director of the disability studies program at the University of Toledo. Her books include *A Disability History of the United States* and *Beyond the Miracle Worker: The Remarkable Life of Anne Sullivan Macy and Her Extraordinary Friendship with Helen Keller*.

Disability Histories

Disability Histories edited by Susan Burch and Michael Rembis
Between Fitness and Death: Disability and Slavery in the Caribbean Stefanie Hunt-Kennedy
Money, Marriage, and Madness: The Life of Anna Ott Kim E. Nielsen

The University of Illinois Press
is a founding member of the
Association of University Presses.

Composed in 10.5/13 Adobe Minion Pro
by Jim Proefrock
at the University of Illinois Press
Cover designed by Charles Brock
Cover illustration: Stanislaw Bohusz-Siestrzencewicz (1869–1927). Portrait study of a sitting woman, early 20th century. National Gallery of Art. Vilnius, Lithuania. (Alamy Stock Photo)

University of Illinois Press
1325 South Oak Street
Champaign, IL 61820-6903
www.press.uillinois.edu